STRENGTH, SPEED & POWER

STRENGTH, SPEED & POWER

Everett Aaberg

ACE, ACSM, CIAR, CSCS, NASM, RTS

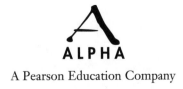

A Pearson Education Company

I dedicate this book to my wife Lane, who has faithfully supported me in this and all my projects.
and in memory of my close friend and mentor Charlie Ragus.

International Standard Book Number: 0-02-864332-1

Library of Congress Catalog Card Number: 2002103788

04 03 02   8 7 6 5 4 3 2 1

Interpretation of the printing code: The rightmost number of the first series of numbers is the year of the book's printing; the rightmost number of the second series of numbers is the number of the book's printing. For example, a printing code of 02-1 shows that the first printing occurred in 2002.

Printed in the United States of America

Note: This publication contains the opinions and ideas of its author. It is intended to provide helpful and informative material on the subject matter covered. It is sold with the understanding that the author and publisher are not engaged in rendering professional services in the book. If the reader requires personal assistance or advice, a competent professional should be consulted.

The author and publisher specifically disclaim any responsibility for any liability, loss, or risk, personal or otherwise, which is incurred as a consequence, directly or indirectly, of the use and application of any of the contents of this book.

Trademarks

All terms mentioned in this book that are known to be or are suspected of being trademarks or service marks have been appropriately capitalized. Alpha Books and Pearson Education, Inc., cannot attest to the accuracy of this information. Use of a term in this book should not be regarded as affecting the validity of any trademark or service mark.

For marketing and publicity, please call: 317-581-3722

The publisher offers discounts on this book when ordered in quantity for bulk purchases and special sales.

For sales within the United States, please contact: Corporate and Government Sales, 1-800-382-3419 or corpsales@pearsontechgroup.com

Outside the United States, please contact: International Sales, 317-581-3793 or international@pearsontechgroup.com

Publisher: Marie Butler-Knight
Product Manager: Phil Kitchel
Managing Editor: Jennifer Chisholm
Acquisitions Editor: Mike Sanders
Development Editor: Michael Koch
Production Editor: Billy Fields
Copy Editor: Rachel Lopez
Cover Designer/Book Designer: Trina Wurst
Creative Director: Robin Lasek
Indexer: Brad Herriman
Layout/Proofreading: Svetlana Dominguez, Stacey Richwine-DeRome

Contents

1   The Human Body: Anatomical Design and Function 1

2   Strength and Endurance, Stability and Mobility 33

3   Agility, Speed, and Power 45

4   Resistance Training Technique 57

5   Strength and Stability Exercises 79

6   Speed, Agility, and Power Exercises 165

7   Progressive Program Design 183

    Bibliography 215

    Index 219

Foreword

Every once in a while a teacher comes along who has a special understanding of the body of knowledge that makes up his or her profession and the ability to make it live for his or her students. Everett Aaberg is one of those rare teachers. His passion for his work is evident in the many aspects of his performance. His conduct, physical bearing, and of course, his training show focus and attention to detail that are reassuring, if you are one of his clients, and awe-inspiring, whether you are an unsophisticated or highly educated observer.

Everett's enthusiasm for discovering and presenting well-documented truths, the most current research, and other essential information on the complex designs of the human body is easy to see. His enthusiasm and discoveries will become obvious to you as you begin reading this book. In addition, he gives principles, techniques, and methods in every chapter on how to improve the body's abilities in its structure and function. Further, clarity of presentation and documentation is supported liberally throughout the book with numerous graphics and references.

Everett's work herein is one of the finest combinations of science and practical instruction that I have ever read. Several sound principles I recognize were pulled from numerous experts' works to lay the foundation for building his unique training techniques and programming concepts. As such, it would seem to me inevitable that with proper application anyone who chooses to follow these methods should see significant progress.

Yet, his continued stress of safety and proper progression keeps this text as a great resource for the beginner as well as the advanced athlete. Improved balance of strength, endurance, joint mobility, and stability, prior to any aggressive training of speed, agility, and power, should be stressed and practiced by more athletic coaches today. The result of such an emphasis would be a reduction in the incidence and severity of injury, besides an increase in athletic performance.

Away from the world of competitive sport, this book is perhaps even more ideal for the personal trainer, fitness enthusiast, and recreational athlete. Aaberg does not dwell on sport-specific programming. Rather, he provides an excellent path for developing the bio-motor abilities of the human body—particularly strength, speed, power, and endurance—so that an increased reservoir of basic elements of athletic performance abilities is developed first. Consequently, these basic elements, for most of us, provide the basic fitness levels essential for activities of daily living. On the other hand, the competitive demands and required skills of professional and elite athletes will obviously need to be integrated into the fine-tuning of the neuromuscular system. In that case, actual game and game-like conditions (sport-specific practices) are the only way to complete their development.

In summary, as a sports scientist, college teacher and coach, Olympic throws coach, and professional football strength and conditioning coach for many years, I have seen my share of philosophies and programs dedicated to the development of increased human performance. During my career, I spent 14 years with the Dallas Cowboys, plus 4 years consulting in the

NFL using sophisticated computer graphics technology to assess on-field playing ability of players. This information confirmed the fact that an NFL player's tenure is determined by his ability to perform through an arduous season and many times at less than 100 percent of his abilities. Injuries during the season can considerably reduce a player's quality of play. Therefore, if a player wanted to have a long career, he had to stay as injury-free as possible and improve his performance as a matter of course. I believe that my experiences, combined with my continued competition as a Masters Competitor and my work in sports research have given me a unique perspective from which to evaluate this book.

In conclusion, I'd like to highly recommend this book for your library and feel confident that those you touch will reap the benefits.

Bob Ward, PED

Director, Sports Science
AdvoCare International
Former Sports Scientist
Strength and Conditioning Coach
Dallas Cowboys 1976–1989

Introduction

Human beings have long searched for methods of improving strength, speed, and power. These precious attributes are the measure of a person's physical abilities and the keys to athletic performance. Being able to run faster, jump higher, or throw farther are crucial to the success of many athletes' careers. However, upon further investigation, you'll find that these abilities are interdependent, as well as dependent on the development of other bio-motor abilities. Strength, stability, mobility, and endurance provide the prerequisite legs that support the fitness base upon which all human performance is built; they are critical for the further development of speed, agility, and power. This fitness base is important not only to the competitive athlete, but to anyone who is interested in increasing the functional use of his or her body for improved quality of daily life.

How This Book Is Organized

This book provides a scientific and systematic approach to proportional development of all the bio-motor abilities that contribute to improved function and optimal performance.

Chapter 1, "The Human Body: Anatomical Design and Function," presents the three major systems responsible, through their coordinated efforts, for any and all human movement. By understanding the major components of the control sensorimotor system, the active muscular system, and the passive-skeletal system, you will understand the relative contributions and the required adaptations of each system necessary for improved performance. This pertinent information on human structure offers valuable insight to improving its function through proper exercise selection, technique, and programming. Understanding the basic interactions of the various systems and subsystems of the body and brain will help you choose and perform the best exercises for the specific goal at the appropriate time.

Chapter 2, "Strength and Endurance, Stability and Mobility," and **Chapter 3, "Speed, Agility, and Power,"** provide you with background information and basic principles for increasing all bio-motor abilities—strength, endurance, stability, mobility, speed, agility, and power. The interdependent relationships and the need to sequentially establish base abilities before focusing on performance abilities will be clearer after reading this.

Chapter 4, "Resistance Training Technique," presents the science behind the development of a safe and efficient exercise technique. These seven elements of technique are critical to achieve maximal results from any resistance training exercise; they also diminish risk of immediate injury and long-term wear. The overall training goals affect and often dictate every other element of technique, so they should be identified before engaging in any resistance training exercise. Learning to evaluate all aspects of the exercise movement such as type, range, speed, and specificity of motion is necessary to develop optimal technique. The alignment, positioning, stabilization demands, and breathing methods are all equally important elements of technique that should also be considered when performing any resistance training exercise.

Chapter 5, "Strength and Stability Exercises," and **Chapter 6, "Speed, Agility, and Power Exercises,"** present the most effective collection of exercises for improving all bio-motor abilities, particularly, strength, speed, and power. All exercises are complete, with detailed instructions and graphics that demonstrate ideal alignment, positioning, motion, and overall technique for optimal efficiency and safety.

Chapter 7, "Progressive Program Design," pulls all previous information together and puts it into action for designing progressive exercise programs and developing a more athletic and functional body. Learning the four major variables and their individual components of exercise programming will empower you to make wiser, more informed decisions on exercise selection and program design. Sample programs that integrate the most effective principles for manipulating program variables for various stages of ability are presented as examples and for trial performance. A periodization model of an exercise program complete with its various cycles and phases is also presented to demonstrate how you can use this valuable system to develop similar models that are more specific to achieving your own needs and training goals.

Whom This Book Is For

This book is designed for the athlete or active person who desires increased strength, speed, power, and overall improved performance of his or her body. It also is a valuable resource for those who train them. This book will increase the efficiency of your training efforts by providing combined information on the structure, functions, and adaptations of the human body with the exercises, techniques, and programs that comprise a system for improving it. By applying this information and the basic training principles presented herein, both overall fitness and performance should be maximized.

How to Use This Book

To best utilize this book to accomplish your fitness and performance goals, or the needs and goals of those you train, I suggest the following protocol. Begin with a study of Chapter 1. This will provide the information upon which all training philosophies, techniques, and programs are based. Continue to occasionally review this chapter and the accompanying figures when designing new programs and selecting different exercises. This might assist you with making better choices and visualizing the specific adaptations you desire for your body.

Familiarize yourself with the training priorities and principles presented in Chapters 2 and 3 that focus on the seven bio-motor abilities of the human body. These chapters offer important guidelines that will influence exercise selection, technique, and programming. Next, look through the various exercises for developing strength and stability in Chapter 5, and the speed, agility, and power exercises in Chapter 6. It is not important or advisable to attempt learning every one of them initially; study only those that might be included in your next program. Master those that were selected, then try a few new exercises for the following program.

Read thoroughly through Chapter 7 to fully understand the interdependent relationships of the major program variables and how to properly adjust them. Begin by designing a base program that focuses on structural development and addresses training needs before being overly concerned with training goals. This should result in a program that is similar to the base program provided in this chapter. Progress to more advanced routines and master each new exercise movement as they come. Eventually, you can begin periodization by designing long-term macrocycles and shorter-term mesocycles that are also presented in this final chapter.

Good luck and God bless.

Acknowledgments

A book such as this is never a product of a single effort, but rather a process entailing numerous years of research, study, and practical experience. And not so much as my own, but that of the numerous experts before me, whose work I cannot re-create, but only build upon. A quick review of the bibliography at the end of this book only recognizes the authors that provided the most critical information used for much of the development of the content presented herein. This in no way represents the hundreds of other researchers, educators, experts, coaches, and mentors whose work has had a profound impact on my presentation of any educational resource. However, there are some that I must acknowledge who have helped me the most thus far in my career.

First, I must thank the Cooper Institute and Dr. Susan Johnson for all their contributions to my professional growth. The opportunity they have provided for me to learn, instruct, and develop resources for such a world-renown research and education organization has given me more credibility than I could have obtained on my own. Their continued support and confidence in me are much appreciated.

I must also recognize physical therapist and biomechanics expert Tom Purvis. His teaching and mentorship have been instrumental in shaping my views on training the human body. His long-time assistance in my education and his friendship have driven my advancement in the fitness industry.

Next, I must thank fitness expert and rehabilitation specialist Paul Chek for his dedication to research and passion for teaching, both of which I have benefited from immensely over the last few years. His abundance of books, videos, courses, and our personal meetings together have directly contributed greatly to the development of content for this book. I look forward to our continued relationship. Charles Poliquin, professional strength coach and friend, has also been an important influence for change in this industry. He has helped me personally with increasing my knowledge base, particularly about the science behind program design and periodization. Mike Clark and the NASM have also been valuable contributors to this industry and my education.

Foremost, I must thank Dr. Robert Ward for his valuable knowledge and information on resistance training science. I am truly honored and humbled to have such an icon of the industry offer to write the foreword for this book. His work as a sports scientist, professional and Olympic strength coach, as well as clinical researcher and author has earned him a reputation as one of the foremost experts in human performance. A special thanks also goes out to Mr. Charlie Ragus and AdvoCare. Without their support and sponsorship, projects like this book would not have been possible for me to pursue.

Last, I would like to thank Pearson Education, Inc., and their staff for the opportunity to share this information with the athletes, coaches, fitness enthusiasts, and trainers who have obtained this book. I hope you are able to learn and progress with its use, as I have in its research and writing.

The Human Body: Anatomical Design and Function

The human body is a highly sophisticated machine uniquely composed of an extremely large but finite number of individual components, which can produce an almost infinite variety of postures and movements.[26] These components are highly integrated and function together as interdependent systems and subsystems. Therefore, if you want to improve the overall performance of the human machine, you should first become familiar with its basic structure and the functions for which it was designed.

This chapter presents a concise and simplified overview of the major systems and subsystems that produce the forces necessary to control all movements of the human body. This chapter also will serve as a reference for anatomical design and joint motion. Muscle *kinematics* will be presented in both the traditional view of isolated *uniplanular* joint motions and in a more functional view that focuses on the coordinated and synergistic actions of the neural, muscular, and skeletal systems.

Several authors and experts have adopted a more contemporary view of anatomy by considering joint and muscle mechanics as they function during the daily movement patterns we perform in our natural environment.[11, 19, 26] This approach differs from the traditional view of anatomy, which typically considered joint motion from a preset, anatomical position. Traditional anatomy also presents all movement as an isolated motion performed in one of the three designated planes. This might be valuable for learning muscle geography (or topography) and relating specific muscles to their appropriate joint movements, but it does not illustrate the integrated muscle actions necessary to perform most activities.

The body can be viewed as being composed of three basic interdependent systems. This model is adopted from Panjabi's studies on segmental spinal stability and has since been utilized by several authors.[15, 19, 36] These three systems are the control or *sensorimotor* system, the active or muscular system, and the passive or skeleton system. These systems must work synergistically for any body or body-segment movement to occur. The following figure shows a schematic representation of these three systems and their interdependent relationships. Each system will be covered in further detail for better understanding of its interdependent role.

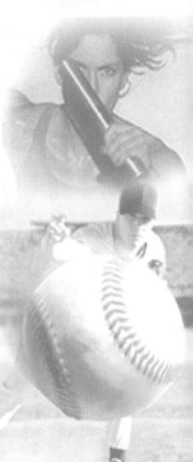

Control / sensorimotor system

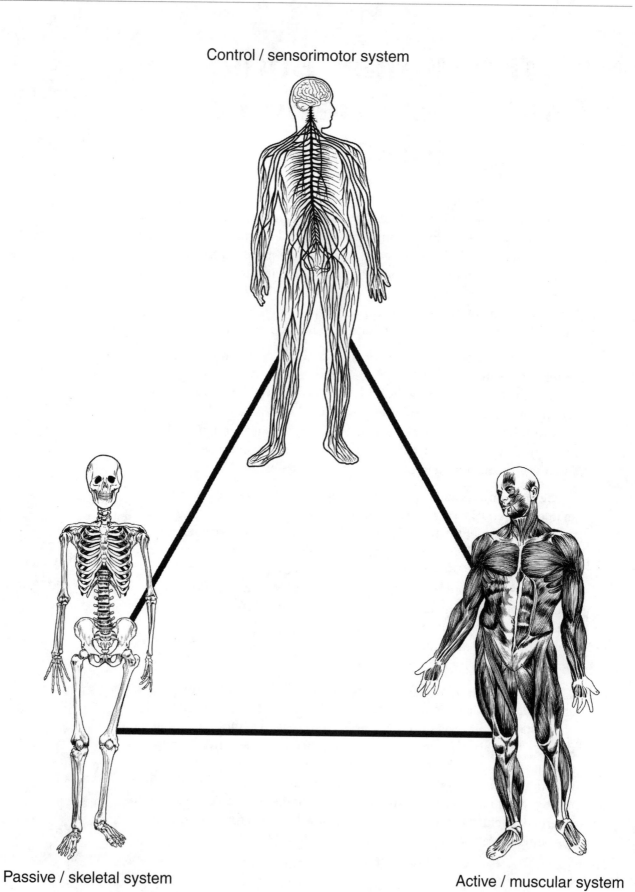

Passive / skeletal system   Active / muscular system

The three systems of human movement.

The Passive System

The passive system is composed of the skeleton, joints, and associated connective tissue. The system is called *passive* because no independent action associated with movement can be accomplished by this system. It is a reactive system that is totally reliant on the forces produced by the active and control systems for movement.

The Skeleton

At birth, the human body is constructed with approximately 270 bones, some of which are designed to fuse as we grow. The adult skeleton normally consists of 206 bones providing a lightweight yet strong, protective, and supportive structure for all other systems of the body. According to Watkins, the skeleton performs three main mechanical functions[42]:

1. It acts as a supportive framework for the rest of the body.
2. It acts as a system of levers on which the muscles can pull in order to stabilize and move the body.
3. It protects certain organs such as the brain, spinal cord, heart, and lungs.

The bones are typically divided into two main groups: the *axial* skeleton and the *appendicular* skeleton. The adult axial skeleton is composed of approximately 80 bones, which form the skull, spine, and rib cage. The axial skeleton provides the foundation for the body and protects the brain, spinal cord, and major organs. Therefore, it is understandable why static and dynamic stabilization of the axial skeleton and pelvis is such a critical element of exercise technique.

The appendicular skeleton is composed of 126 bones, which make up the scapula and upper limbs, as well as the pelvis and lower limbs. All human movement other than spinal motion is a result of synergistic muscle pulls on the appendicular skeleton. This collection of bones provides the lever systems that enable us to exert force against our environment in order to move the body or any external objects.

The following figure details the construction of the human skeleton for easy reference.

The Joints

The bones are held together by joints and associated connective tissue, which are not pictured in the figure on the following page but are vital components of the passive-skeletal system. Each joint of the body is specifically constructed to allow and limit movement of the bones at their attachments. There are three structural classifications of joints, each with distinct levels of possible articulation:

* **Fibrous joints** allow for very little, if any, movement because of the small amount of space between bone endings. They include the joints of the skull, the joints between the radius and ulna of the lower arm, and the distal connection of the fibula and tibia of the lower leg.

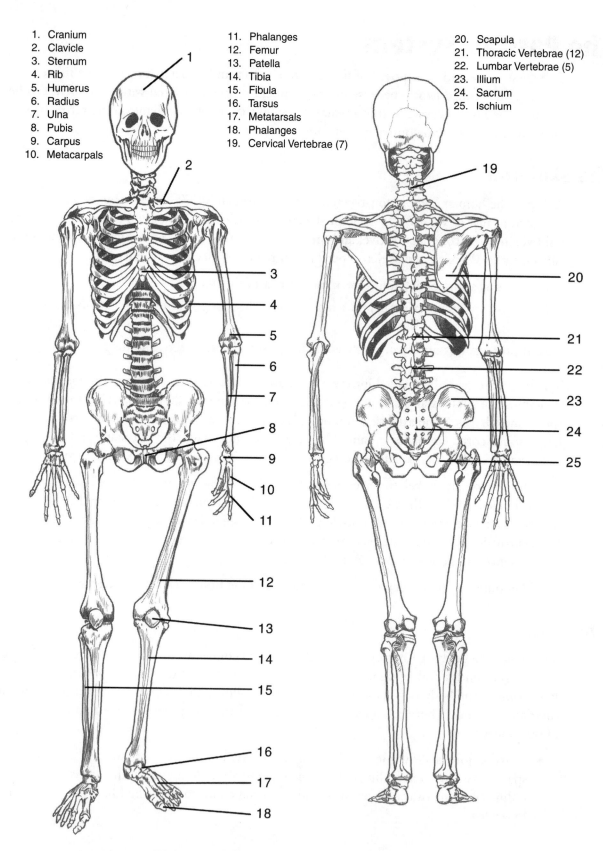

1. Cranium
2. Clavicle
3. Sternum
4. Rib
5. Humerus
6. Radius
7. Ulna
8. Pubis
9. Carpus
10. Metacarpals

11. Phalanges
12. Femur
13. Patella
14. Tibia
15. Fibula
16. Tarsus
17. Metatarsals
18. Phalanges
19. Cervical Vertebrae (7)

20. Scapula
21. Thoracic Vertebrae (12)
22. Lumbar Vertebrae (5)
23. Illium
24. Sacrum
25. Ischium

The passive-skeletal system—front and back view of skeleton.

* **Cartilaginous joints** allow for limited capacities of movement because of their proportionally higher collagen-to-elastin fiber compositions. Examples of cartilaginous joints would be those that connect the ribs to the sternum and the intervertebral disks of the spine. Although both fibrous and cartilaginous joints serve specific and highly important functions, a book dealing with human movement would be most concerned with the joint structures that offer more freedom for movement.[26]

* **Synovial joints** account for most of the joints of the human body; each is individually designed with a considerable variance for range of motion. There are three types of synovial joints, categorized by the number of directions in which they can rotate around their given axis—uniaxial, biaxial, and multiaxial joints; these are depicted in the following figures.

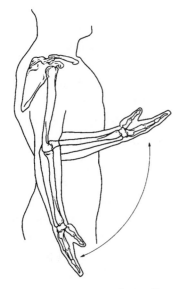

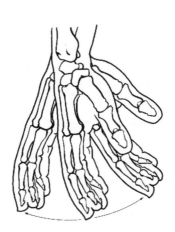

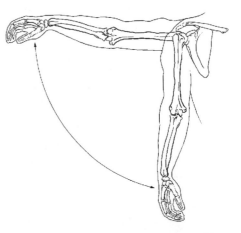

Uniaxial joints *have only one direction of rotation and operate much like a hinge. The elbow and the phalangeal joints of the fingers are examples.*

Biaxial joints *such as the wrist, ankle, and knee (when flexed) allow for movement in two perpendicular planes.*

Multiaxial joints *such as the shoulder and hip allow for movement in all three planes of motion to provide us with the largest degrees and varieties of possible movement.*

Passive Connective Tissue

A joint's capacity for movement is determined only in part by the structure and congruence of the bones themselves. Connective tissues hold the bones together and regulate the type, direction, and range of motion between the bone endings. The two major types of connective tissues in synovial joints are ligaments and joint capsules. These serve as the passive, noncontractile links between the bone endings, where larger degrees of movement are designed to take place.

* **Ligaments** connect bone to bone and consist primarily of strong collagen fibers arranged parallel to each other with only small amounts of elastic fiber. They are designed to restrict joint movement to specific directions and specific ranges of movement. They are not capable of any significant stretching without deformation or tearing. Ligaments can

be a part of the joint capsule or separate; they can be located inside or outside the capsule, depending on the designed function of the joint and its needs for mobility and stability.[42]

* **Joint capsules** enclose the joint, creating a cavity that holds fluid in the joint and helps to transfer forces from bone to bone. The capsule typically is composed of two or more layers of regular collagenous tissue, which form a sleeve around the joint. The parallel collagen fiber arrangements of each layer typically are laid down at different angles to the adjacent layers. This enables the capsule to allow for joint movement in several directions, while also assisting with joint stability.[42]

Cartilage is another substance found at synovial joints that should also be considered when analyzing joint movement.

* **Hyaline,** or **articular cartilage,** is a shiny, slick protective covering of bone endings at synovial joints that assists with joint movement. Although articular cartilage is well constructed to absorb some levels of shock and friction, it can be damaged from excessive pressure or mechanical wear, or when movement exceeds designed limits. This is of particular concern when movement is performed under high-impact forces or with heavy external loads. Rheumatoid and osteoarthritis are two common diseases involving damage to articular cartilage that, once begun, often continues to deteriorate joint surfaces, causing inflammation and pain.[10]

* **Fibrocartilage** contains high concentrations of collagenous fibers and is specially designed for absorbing shock. It is a thick, rubber-like material found in the vertebral disks of the spine, menisci of the knee, the pubis symphysis of the pelvis, and other joints in need of the extra cartilage support between bone surfaces. Although resilient, fibrocartilage also is susceptible to thinning, tearing, folding, and rupturing under high levels, or frequent exposure to impact forces and friction. The body's natural replacement of fibrocartilage is limited, which often leaves the joint with little or no disk substance and painful, inefficient joint movement.

Bone structure, congruence, connective tissue, and cartilage all affect joint stability and mobility. As such, you must consider these passive components when performing certain exercise techniques, particularly when determining the optimal range of motion. I will present these issues and similar anatomical factors as they relate to exercise technique in Chapter 4, "Resistance Training Technique."

The Active System

The passive system can preset type, direction, and range of motion but all movement is totally dependent on the muscular, or active, system through the commands delivered by the control system. The muscles of the body are the powerhouses for movement and the link between the control and passive systems. In fact, the interdependent functions of the muscles with both the passive and control systems, gives rise to the classification of two larger combined systems. The *musculoskeletal system* is the combination of the passive and active systems and their synergistic functions.

Likewise, the *neuromuscular system* can be viewed as the combination of the control and active systems and their synergistic functions. The following figures depict these combinations of systems for easier reference, because both terms will be used at times throughout this book.

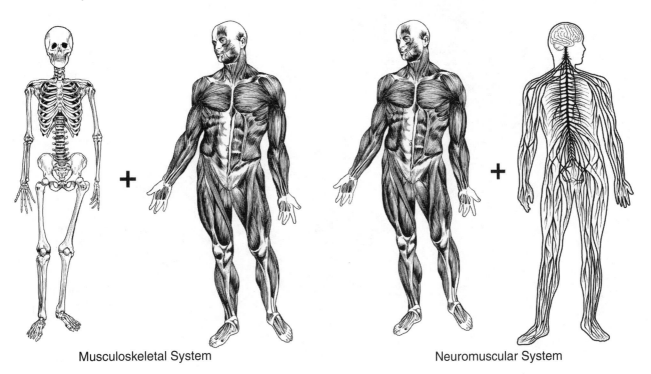

| Musculoskeletal System | Neuromuscular System |

Musculoskeletal system = Passive system + Active system.   *Neuromuscular system = Control system + Active system.*

Basic Muscle Structure and Function

The unique physiological properties of muscles enable them to respond to the commands sent from the control system and immediately produce the appropriate pulling forces that are then applied to the levers of the passive system. These forces serve to position, stabilize, and move the body. The following figure illustrates the physiological structure of a typical *fusiform* muscle-tendon unit for better understanding of muscle function.

Muscles are attached or anchored to the bone through strong fibrous cords known as *tendons*. Each muscle is wrapped in a protective sheath and held together by deep *fascia* called the *epimysium*. Internally, the muscle consists of bundles of muscle fibers called *fasciculi*, which also are wrapped in a protective sheath called the *perimysium*. Inside the fasciculi are the muscle fibers that run the full length of the muscle from origin to insertion and range from a few inches to more than three feet in length.[8]

Muscle fibers are also wrapped in their own protective fascia called the *endomysium*. This deep fascia helps with force production and allows for smooth sliding of adjacent fibers as the muscle lengthens and shortens. Fascia also discourages the development of adhesions between the adjacent fibers that can limit muscle function and cause pain. Inside each muscle fiber are the *myofibrils* that contain the contractile protein filaments known as *myosin* and *actin*. This is where the actual muscle contraction is made possible.

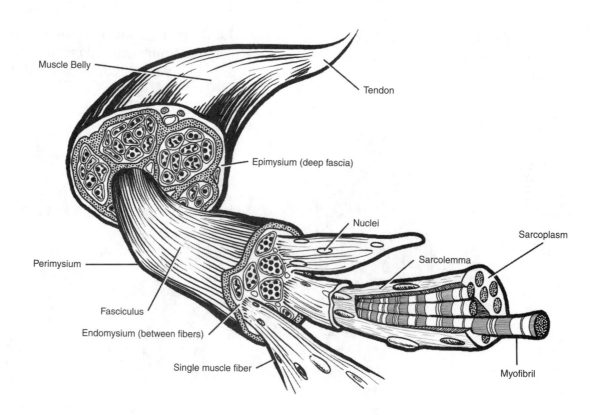

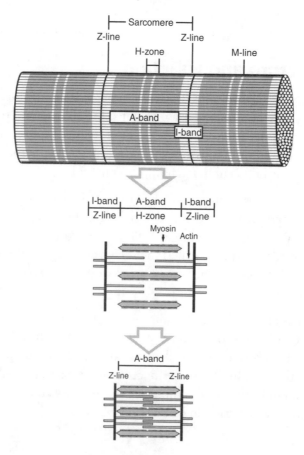

Myofibril

The muscle-tendon unit.

When a muscle is stimulated through a signal from its specific motor unit, a series of chemical reactions involving calcium and ATP takes place, which results in a mechanical pulling action of the actin filaments across the myosin. This sliding effect of the filaments pulls the Z-lines closer together, shortening each *sarcomere* of the muscle fiber, which therefore shortens or contracts the entire muscle. This is the basic process involved in muscle contraction.[10]

Through this same process, a muscle can perform different types of classified contractions. A *concentric contraction* is one in which the muscle-tendon unit is shortening while contracting. An *eccentric contraction* is when the muscle-tendon unit is not producing enough force to shorten and actually is lengthening while contracting. An *isometric contraction* is one in which the muscle-tendon unit is neither shortening nor lengthening, while still producing tension and a contractile force. Any exercise involves all three phases of muscle contraction for each repetition performed.

Aside from their active capabilities to contract, muscles also have passive elastic properties that allow them to tend to return to resting length when tension is removed. They also have passive plastic properties that resist being stretched too far. In fact, plastic properties of the muscle fascia can contribute to more than 40 percent of a joint's level of stiffness or flexibility.[6] With proper stretching and active lengthening techniques, you can reduce some of this resistance through safe adaptations of the fascia. Consequently, repetitive inefficient stretching, ballistic stretching, or forced passive lengthening can cause deformation of the fascia or connective tissues and damage to the muscle. This may alter length-tension relationships and force output, as well as result in overall instability of the joint.

Muscles produce the most force at or just slightly longer than resting length.[8] Contractile force diminishes when the muscle length is significantly shortened or lengthened before contraction. This is because the myosin and actin filaments are already overlapped when significantly shortened, or unable to cross-bridge effectively when significantly lengthened. Either scenario will drastically reduce muscle force and is referred to as *active insufficiency*. Active insufficiency can be described as a muscle's diminished capability to produce active tension or force.[26]

Isolated Joint Kinematics

Any life movement requires the coordinated functions of the control, active, and passive systems. Daily activities rarely include any isolated joint motions performed in a singular plane. An entire concert of integrated neural and muscle actions takes place in order to stabilize joints, neutralize undesired movements, and maintain center of gravity over the base of support during even the most common of daily tasks. For these reasons, study of isolated joint movement is sometimes excluded in contemporary literature dealing with functional anatomy. However, I have found it extremely helpful for fitness professionals and athletes to have a solid understanding of basic muscle mechanics. Knowing which muscles are directly involved in producing the various joint motions of the body assists with efficient exercise selection and basic program design. Even the most complex athletic movements can be eventually broken down to specific combinations of individual joint motions. This enables us to identify possible weak links in the kinetic chain that may be targeted for isolated strengthening in order to improve overall performance.

Movement of the body is traditionally presented as occurring in one of the three basic planes of movement. All joints are assumed to be working in an isolated manner and begin from the anatomical position. The figure on this page depicts the three general planes of joint motion.

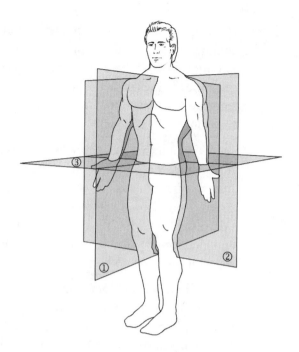

The body can be divided into three perpendicular planes of movement.

* **Plane 1** is the median plane, also known as the *sagital* plane. This plane divides the body down the middle into left and right halves. Most human movement takes place predominantly in the median plane. The joint motions of flexion and extension are the primary movements of the median plane and occur at the ankle, knee, hip, spine, shoulder, elbow, and wrist. Scapular protraction and retraction also are considered median plane movements.

* **Plane 2** is known as the frontal plane and sometimes is presented as the *coronal* plane. This plane divides the body through the side into front and back halves. Joint movements of abduction; adduction of the wrist, shoulder, and hip; and inversion and eversion of the ankle, scapular elevation, depression, upward rotation, downward rotation, and trunk lateral flexion of the spine all are frontal plane movements.

* **Plane 3** is the horizontal plane, also referred to as the *transverse* plane. Internal and external rotation of the knee, hip, and shoulder; the horizontal flexion and extension of the shoulder, *supination*, and *pronation* of the elbow and ankle; and all spinal rotation are considered movements of the horizontal plane. (Supination and pronation of the ankle are special movements requiring combined ankle extension with inversion and combined ankle flexion with eversion, respectively. Supination and pronation of the ankle are coupled with hip, pelvic, and resulting spinal positions, which dramatically affect posture and overall movement abilities of the body.)

All individual joint movements occurring in any one of these three general planes can be defined and linked with a specific group of muscles that synergetically produce each motion. The following figures depict the major joint movements of the body. The associated muscle groups that are either prime movers or assistors for the isolated joint movement are listed next to each graphic. Learning this information is helpful, because this terminology is often used to describe human movement. This section will also serve as a quick reference for matching muscles to joint movements.

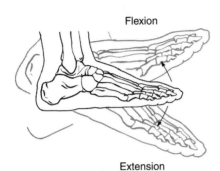

Flexion

Extension

Ankle Flexion
(dorsiflexion)

- tibialis anterior
- extensor halluces longus
- extensor digitorum longus
- peroneus tertius

Ankle Extension
(plantar flexion)

- peroneus longus
- peroneus brevis
- triceps surae
- flexor halluces longus
- tibialis posterior
- flexor digitorum longus

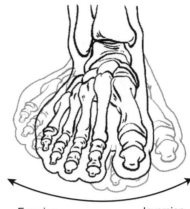

Eversion   Inversion

Ankle Eversion
(partial pronation)

- peroneus longus
- peroneus brevis
- peroneus tertius
- extensor digitorum longus (lateral portion)

Ankle Inversion
(partial supination)

- extensor halluces longus
- tibialis anterior
- tibialis posterior
- flexor digitorum longus
- flexor halluces longus
- triceps surae

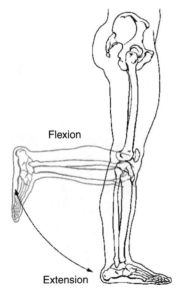

Flexion

Extension

Knee Flexion

- biceps femoris (long & short heads)
- semitendinosus
- semimembranosus
- popliteus
- gastrocnemius
- sartorius
- gracilis

Knee Extension

- vastus lateralis
- vastus medialis
- vastus intermedius
- rectus femoris
- tensor fasciae latae
- gluteus maximus (superficial portion)

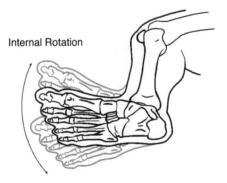

Internal Rotation

External Rotation

Knee Internal Rotation
(medial rotation)

- sartorius
- semitendinosus
- semimembranosus
- gracilis
- popliteus

Knee External Rotation
(lateral rotation)

- tensor fasciae latae
- gluteus maximus (superficial portion)
- biceps femoris (long head)
- biceps femoris (short head)

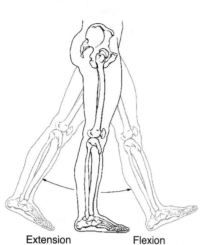

Extension   Flexion

Hip Extension

- gluteus maximus
- biceps femoris (long head)
- semimembranosus
- semitendinosus
- gluteus medius (posterior portion)
- adductor magnus

Hip Flexion

- psoas
- iliacus
- rectus femoris
- tensor fasciae latae
- gluteus minimus and medius (anterior portions)
- sartorius
- pectineus
- gracilis

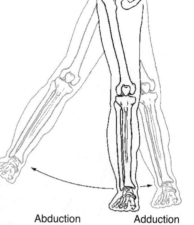

Abduction   Adduction

Hip Abduction

- gluteus medius
- gluteus minimus
- tensor fasciae latae
- gluteus maximus (superficial portion)
- piriformis
- obturators
- gemelli
- sartorius

Hip Adduction

- adductor magnus
- adductor longus
- adductor brevis
- pectineus
- gracilis
- psoas
- iliacus

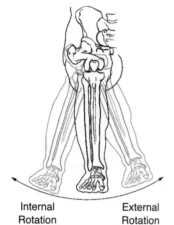

Internal Rotation   External Rotation

Hip Internal Rotation (medial rotation)

- gluteus medius
- gluteus minimus
- tensor fasciae latae

Hip External rotation (lateral rotation)

- gluteus maximus
- gluteus minimus
- piriformis
- obturators
- gemelli
- quadratus femoris
- biceps femoris (long head)

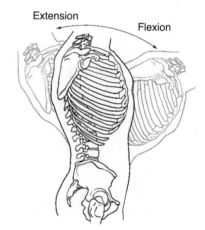

Extension   Flexion

Trunk Extension

- spinalis group
- longissimus group
- iliocostalis group
- transversospinalis group
- interspinalis

Trunk Flexion

- rectus abdominus
- external obliques (bilateral contraction)
- internal obliques (bilateral contraction)

Lateral Flexion

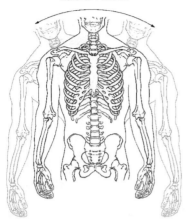

Trunk Lateral Flexion

- internal oblique (unilateral contraction)
- quadratus lumborum (unilateral contraction)
- rectus abdominus (unilateral contraction)
- erector spinae groups (unilateral contraction)
- latissimus dorsi (unilateral contraction)
- transversospinalis group (unilateral contraction)
- intertransverse (unilateral contraction)

Depression

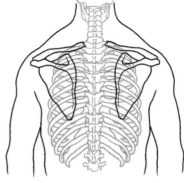

Scapular Depression

- lower trapezius
- lower serratus anterior
- pectoralis minor
- subclavius (via the clavicle)

Elevation

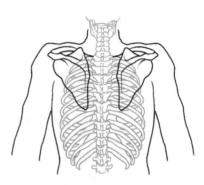

Scapular Elevation

- levator scapulae
- upper trapezius
- rhomboids

Rotation

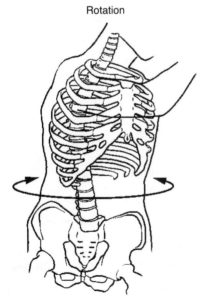

Trunk Rotation

- erector spinae groups (unilateral contraction)
- transversospinalis group (unilateral contraction)
- external obliques (unilateral contraction)
- internal oblique (contralateral contraction)

Protraction

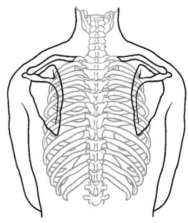

Scapular Protraction (abduction)

- mid serratus anterior
- upper serratus anterior (superior)
- lower serratus anterior (inferior)

Retraction

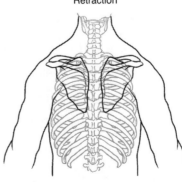

Scapular Retraction (adduction)

- mid trapezius
- rhomboids
- lower trapezius
- upper trapezius

Downward Rotation

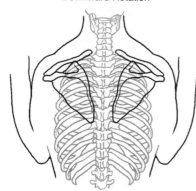

Scapular Downward Rotation

- rhomboids
- levator scapulae

Upward Rotation

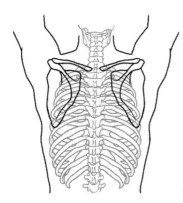

Scapular Upward Rotation

- upper trapezius
- lower trapezius
- upper serratus anterior (superior)

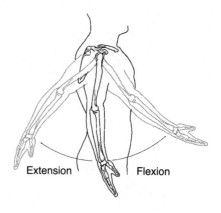

Extension   Flexion

Shoulder Extension

- latissimus dorsi
- posterior deltoid
- teres minor

Shoulder Flexion

- anterior deltoid
- pectoralis major
- coracobrachialis

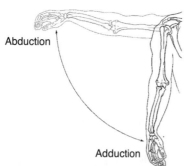

Abduction

Adduction

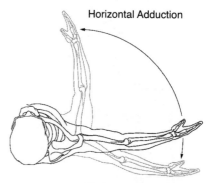

Horizontal Adduction

Horizontal Abduction

Shoulder Abduction

- deltoid
- supraspinatus
- infraspinatus (accessory)
- long head biceps (accessory)
- upper subscapularis (accessory)

Shoulder Adduction

- latissimus dorsi
- pectoralis major
- teres major
- teres minor (accessory)

Shoulder Horizontal Adduction

- pectoralis major (sternal)
- pectoralis major (clavicular)
- anterior deltoid
- coracobrachialis (accessory)
- biceps brachii (accessory)

Shoulder Horizontal Abduction

- posterior deltoid
- infraspinatus
- teres minor
- scapular retractors (accessory)

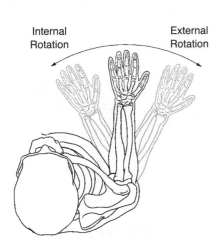

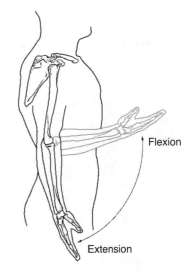

Shoulder Internal Rotation (medial rotation)

- subscapularis
- latissimus dorsi
- pectoralis major
- teres major
- anterior deltoid

Shoulder External Rotation (lateral rotation)

- infraspinatus
- teres minor
- posterior deltoid

Elbow Extension

- triceps (long head)
- triceps (lateral head)
- triceps medial head (deep head)
- anconeus

Elbow Flexion

- biceps brachii
- brachioradialis
- brachialis

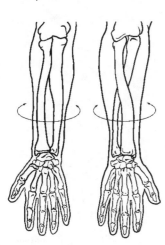

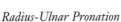

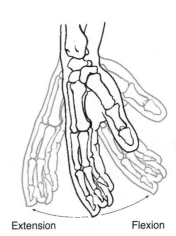

Radius-Ulnar Supination

- biceps brachii
- supinator

Radius-Ulnar Pronation

- pronator teres
- pronator quadratus
- brachioradialis

Wrist Extension

- extensor carpi radialis longus
- extensor carpi radialis brevis
- extensor carpi ulnaris

Wrist Flexion

- flexor carpi radialis
- palmaris longus
- flexor carpi ulnaris

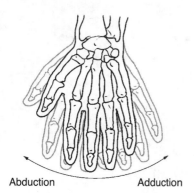

Abduction   Adduction

Wrist Abduction

- flexor carpi radialis
- extensor carpi radialis longus
- extensor carpi radialis brevis

Wrist Adduction

- flexor carpi ulnaris
- extensor carpi ulnaris

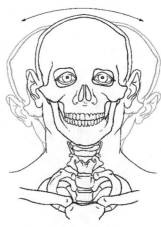

Lateral Flexion

Neck Lateral Flexion

- scalenus group (unilateral contraction)
- sternocleidomastoid (unilateral contraction)
- longus colli (unilateral contraction)
- rectus capitis (unilateral contraction)
- longus capitis (unilateral contraction)
- splenius capitis (unilateral contraction)
- splenius cervicis (unilateral contraction)
- spinalis capitis (unilateral contraction)
- semispinalis capitis (unilateral contraction)
- trapezius (unilateral contraction)

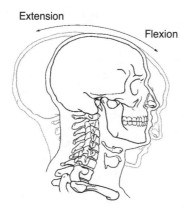

Extension   Flexion

Neck Flexion

- longus colli (bilateral contraction)
- rectus capitis (bilateral contraction)
- longus capitis (bilateral contraction)
- sternocleidomastoid (bilateral contraction)
- suprahyoid group (accessory)
- infrahyoid group (accessory)

Neck Extension

- splenius capitis (bilateral contraction)
- splenius cervicis (bilateral contraction)
- spinalis capitis (bilateral contraction)*
- semispinalis capitis (bilateral contraction)*
- spinalis thoracis
- levator scapulae (bilateral contraction)
- trapezius (bilateral contraction)

*when spine is fixed or stabilized

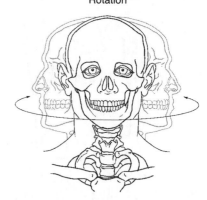

Rotation

Neck Rotation

- sternocleidomastoid (unilateral contraction)*
- trapezius (unilateral contraction)*
- longus colli (unilateral contraction)
- rectus capitis (unilateral contraction)
- splenius capitis (unilateral contraction)
- splenius cervicis (unilateral contraction)
- spinalis capitis (unilateral contraction)
- semispinalis capitis (unilateral contraction)

*contralateral rotation

Muscle Actions and Roles

Although muscles can dominate one plane of motion, the control system is designed to coordinate muscle synergies and recruits muscles for a variety of functions. Depending on the load, the direction of resistance, and body positioning, muscles can play different roles, such as *agonists, antagonists, synergists, stabilizers,* or *neutralizers.*[19]

* **Agonists** are muscles that act as prime movers for the desired motion. The agonists are not only responsible for accelerating the concentric movement, they also decelerate the eccentric portion of the movement and perform isometric contraction as well. For example, the biceps muscle group accelerates elbow flexion, decelerates elbow extension, and can isometrically help to stabilize the elbow at any point of loaded biceps movement.

* **Antagonists** are the muscles that work in direct opposition to the present movement. To contract any muscle, the opposing muscle must release most of its tension through an action known as *reciprocal inhibition.* Complete inhibition of a properly functioning muscle is highly unlikely as mechanoreceptors are always monitoring and assisting with control of muscle tension for protection and operation of the joint. Antagonists are also needed for deceleration during fast concentric movements, such as throwing a ball or swinging a bat.[25]

* **Synergists** are muscles that assist the agonists, or prime movers, with their concentric movements. The degree of assistance they offer depends on the amount of load, direction of resistance, and the overall capabilities of the primary movers. For example, if the glutes are inhibited for some reason, more assistance from the hamstrings will be recruited to perform hip extension, and possibly more assistance from the piriformis will be required for performing external rotation.

  If the inhibition of any muscle becomes pronounced enough or chronic, associated synergists will always attempt to compensate, which leads to a condition known as *synergistic dominance.*[19] This condition of compensation can cause further alterations in muscle length-tension relationships, which can affect posture, limit performance, or reduce overall joint integrity.

* **Stabilizers** are muscles that isometrically (or quasi-isometrically) hold a certain joint position or govern the joint's overall movement. Muscles designed for stabilization, such as the deep postural muscles of spine, are referred to as *tonic muscles.* Tonic muscles are constructed for endurance, have low force output, and almost always function as stabilizers. However, *phasic muscles* can also act as stabilizers when needed. Stabilization is a critical role for muscles to perform, and must always precede movement.

* **Neutralizers** are muscles that exert light forces to counteract an unwanted action of another muscle. For example, certain core muscles, such as the multifidi, work in concert with the psoas and erector spinea to neutralize shearing forces at the lumbar spine. Without proper functioning of neutralizers, joint mechanics are altered and faulty motor patterns develop, which can cause compensation and an increased incidence of injury or joint degeneration.[19]

The following figure illustrates the active-muscular system. This will be helpful for learning muscle location and better visualization of basic muscle function. By simply observing the general direction of fiber alignment of any muscle, you can easily see how it will exert a pull on the limb or torso to produce a specific movement or to stabilize against external forces. For example, the general orientation of the pectoralis fibers run predominantly at a horizontal angle. Therefore, it is a logical deduction that exercises resisting horizontal adduction (also known as horizontal flexion) would be the best alignment to target this musculature.

1. Platysma
2. Deltoid
3. Pectoralis major
4. Biceps brachii
5. Pronator teres
6. Flexor group
7. External oblique
8. Rectus abdominus
9. Adductors
10. Sartorius
11. Rectus femoris
12. Vastus medialis
13. Peroneus longus
14. Tibialis anterior
15. Coracobrachialis
16. Brachialis
17. Internal oblique
18. Brachioradialis
19. Flexor digitorum superficialis

20. Trapezius
21. Deltoid
22. Triceps brachii
23. Latissimus dorsi
24. Extensor group
25. Gluteus maximus
26. Iliotibial tract
27. Biceps femoris
28. Semitendinosus

29. Gastrocnemius
30. Splenius capitis
31. Levator scapula
32. Rhomboids
33. Infraspinatus
34. Teres minor
35. Teres major
36. Erector spinae
37. Serratus posterior inferior
38. Gluteus minimus
39. Gluteus medius (cut)
40. Piriformis
41. Semimembranosus
42. Plantaris
43. Popliteus
44. Soleus

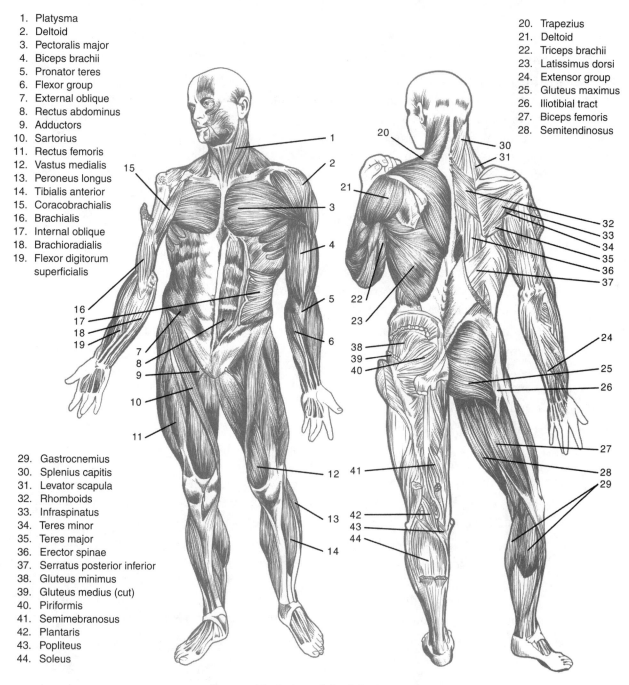

Front and back views of the skeletal muscles.

Active-Muscular Subsystems

When viewing anatomy as an active integrated system, we find that muscles never work in isolation. In fact, we rarely even attempt to perform any isolated joint movements in life outside of our traditional gym exercises. The control system does not typically recruit individual muscles for isolated joint motion, but rather activates muscle groups that synergistically work to stabilize, neutralize, accelerate, and decelerate the body as it moves in any or all three planes.[19]

Research has identified several muscular subsystems the body regularly uses for stabilization and movement during general movement patterns. The subsystems and functions most pertinent to improving bio-motor capabilities are …

* The inner unit
* The deep longitudinal subsystem
* The posterior oblique subsystem
* The anterior oblique subsystem
* The lateral subsystem

A brief summary of each of these subsystems is provided to help you understand each of their interdependent roles in various movements. This insight to some of the body's integrated muscle actions should help in exercise selections and for designing more effective training programs. You will also notice that certain exercises and techniques presented in this book are specifically intended to strengthen these various subsystems rather than target individual muscles. I'll begin with the *inner unit*.

The Inner Unit (The Core)

Several authors have cited research on spinal segmental stabilization that has clearly identified a local stabilizing system known as the inner unit.[10, 14, 19] This deep layer of abdominal, pelvic, and spinal musculature provides dual functions of respiration and stabilization. The inner unit is uniquely designed to accomplish both tasks simultaneously when working properly and is under separate neurological control from the outer trunk muscles such as the rectus abdominus, external obliques, and some of the erector spinea muscles.[12]

Because of this separate neural relationship and its unique roles, the inner unit will be referred to as the "core." The outer abdominal, oblique, and spinal muscles will be referred to simply as "trunk" muscles. This distinct use of the word "core" to specifically represent the inner unit and to delineate it from the outer layers of trunk musculature is for teaching purposes only. Most authors typically use the words "core" and "trunk" synonymously. There is nothing wrong with this popular view, as the entire midsection of the body is constructed of overlapping layers of muscle, which work in concert with each other to perform both stability and movement actions to meet a variety of demands. However, in my own experience as a lecturer, author, and trainer, I have found it easier to discuss the unique functions of the inner unit and teach techniques for strengthening it by verbally separating the core from the outer-trunk muscles.

The inner unit or core is composed of superior, inferior, anterior, and posterior muscles that enclose the contents of the abdominal cavity, or viscera. The primary muscles of the core are the diaphragm, the pelvic floor muscles, the transverse abdominus, and the multifidi. However, posterior fibers of the internal obliques, the quadratus lumborum, the intertransversari, interspinales, and other deep spinal erector muscles also assist with core functions, particularly when it comes to stabilization. All these muscles attach to a large, broad, and flattened tendon called an *aponeurosis*. This particular aponeurosis is referred to most often as the *thoracolumbar fascia*.[40]

The thoracolumbar fascia is a network of noncontractile tissue divided into three layers: anterior, middle, and posterior.[12, 36, 42] It plays a vital role in spinal stabilization and provides a critical force-transference mechanism for the various muscular subsystems of the body. With the assistance of the thoracolumbar fascia the core muscles help to provide intra-abdominal pressure to stabilize the spine while still performing respiratory functions.[20, 36] The following figure demonstrates the stabilization actions of the inner unit during respiration.

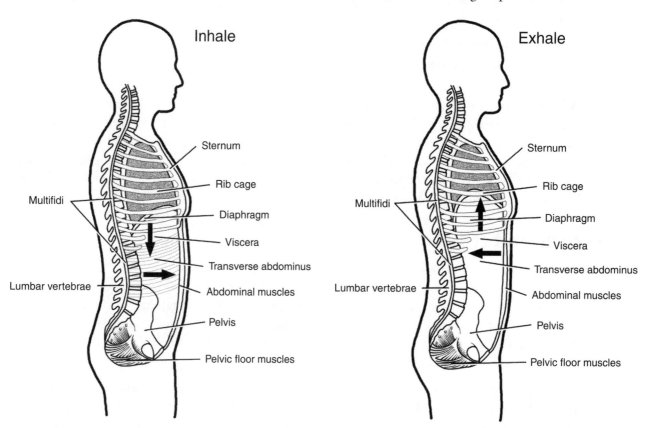

The inner unit, or core.

Upon inhalation, unrestricted diaphragm contraction creates a downward pull on the contents of the abdominal cavity, simultaneously helping the lungs to draw in more air and expand the thoracic cavity. This downward force pushes the viscera down against the bowl of the pelvis, which signals a co-contraction of the pelvic floor muscles. The viscera also presses forward, causing a slight distension of the abdominal wall, which creates passive tension from the transverse abdominus and a tightening of the thoracolumbar fascia. This, combined with the simultaneous backward pressure of the viscera, assists the multifidi and deep erector muscles to create a stiffening of the spine. At full inhalation both cavities are pressurized; by simply holding the breath and tightening abdominal muscles we create the *Valsalva Maneuver*—a stabilization technique of the spine that can be done purposefully or through a reflex action—thus achieving maximal stability of the spine.

The greater challenge for spinal and postural stabilization occurs when exhaling, because pressure can be reduced in both the abdominal and thoracic cavities. However, through a contraction of the transverse abdominus this pressure loss is minimized and the resulting core activation assists with continued stabilization. The contraction of the transverse abdominus creates a drawing-in of the viscera, much like the tightening of a belt. This presses the viscera back, down, and upward, which is coupled with co-contractions of the pelvic floor muscles, multifidi, associated deep erector muscles, the posterior fibers of the internal oblique, and a reciprocal relaxation of the diaphragm. This maintains pressure in the abdominal and thoracic cavities while assisting with exhalation. During any prolonged resistance training exercise or when lifting any heavy object, this stabilization process is maximized through these described voluntary activations of the transverse abdominus combined with the proper breathing technique. More information pertaining to core activation and breathing techniques will be presented in Chapter 4. Actual core training exercises are also provided in the first section of Chapter 5, "Strength and Stability Exercises." Mastering these exercises will enable you to better integrate proper core activation and breathing into practically every other exercise you perform.

This control of intra-abdominal pressure is believed to be an automated action during the lower-level stabilization demands we encounter in most of our daily activities.[20] A properly functioning core has proven to be the first recruited muscular system before any movement the body performs. This automated reflex action is believed to occur due to the continual need for spinal stabilization and maintenance of center of gravity. Stability is always a prerequisite for movement. However, many experts believe this automated action can become inhibited through injury, surgery, or poor exercise and breathing habits.[11, 19, 36] It is also believed that through proper training, core activation can become an enhanced reflexive action that increases overall neuromuscular efficiency and performance while reducing risk of future injury. Although the core is the critical local stabilization system for the spine, you also need the global muscle subsystems to assist with gross stabilization and provide for movement of the limbs. These subsystems, often referred to as *slings*, attach the trunk to the legs and wrap the pelvic-lumbar area from different angles. They are designed to work in a synergistic manner to produce force couples that provide for optimal control over the lumbar, pelvic, and hip complex.

The Deep Longitudinal Subsystem

The *deep longitudinal subsystem* (DLS) provides for reciprocal force transmission from the ground to the trunk and back down. The DLS includes the tibialis anterior, peroneus longus, biceps femoris, sacrotuberous ligament, erector spinae, and thoracolumbar fascia. This subsystem's major roles are to absorb and transfer ground force and resulting kinetic energy, stabilize the ankle, decelerate forward leg movement, and stabilize the spine by resisting trunk flexion. You can better visualize this system in action as it would function when running by studying the figure on top of the following page.

As the leg moves forward during the swing phase when running, the hamstring muscles activate to decelerate the forward leg movement, or hip flexion and knee extension. The activation of the biceps femoris increases tension in the sacrotuberous ligament, which transfers force across the sacrum; this stabilizes the S.I. joint of the pelvis and allows for force transference up through the erector spinea to also help stabilize the trunk. The action of the biceps femoris also causes tension through the peroneus longus, which works in concert with the anterior tibialis to stabilize the ankle in preparation for the heel to strike the ground. Upon heel strike, resulting ground forces and kinetic energy are captured in the thoracolumbar fascia and later used by the posterior oblique system for the propulsion phase of gait.[12, 19] A dumbbell one-leg hip extension or a barbell hip extension are sample exercises to target the DLS.

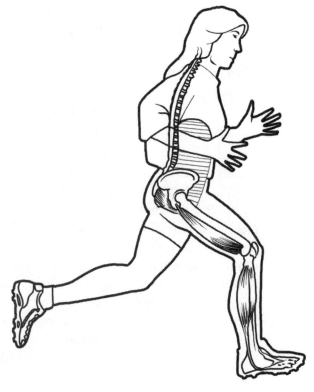

The deep longitudinal subsystem.

The Posterior Oblique Subsystem

The posterior oblique subsystem (POS) is comprised primarily of the latissimus dorsi and the contralateral gluteus. It works synergistically with the DLS through its shared use of the connective thoracolumbar fascia. The POS while running is also demonstrated in action in the following figure.

As the leg moves forward in the swing phase of running, the ipsilateral gluteus maximus assists the hamstrings to decelerate hip flexion, while the contralateral latissimus dorsi activates to decelerate forward flexion of the arm. There is a parallel alignment of the muscle fibers of the gluteus maximus and the contralateral latissimus dorsi. They transfer force across the S.I. joint at a perpendicular angle, which assists to stabilize the pelvis during the impact of heel strike and prepares the entire lumbar-pelvic region for propulsion.

The thoracolumbar fascia then transfers stored kinetic energy to the POS, which in turn accelerates or pulls the arm and opposite leg back, which propels the body forward. The timing of the co-contraction of the POS produces tension that again is transferred to the thoracolumbar fascia. This tension assists with continued pelvic

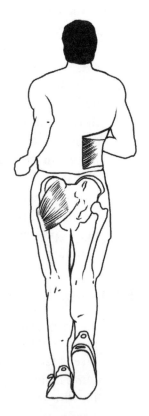

The posterior oblique subsystem.

and lumbar stabilization, and can be stored for use in the following phases of running or gait, which reduces the metabolic cost. The POS also is of prime importance in rotational actions such as swinging a bat or golf club, or when throwing a baseball.[12, 19] A cable one-arm low row performed in a lunge position is a sample exercise to target the POS.

The Anterior Oblique Subsystem

The *anterior oblique subsystem* (AOS) works similarly to the POS, only from an anterior orientation. The AOS is composed primarily of the adductors of the hip with their ipsilateral internal obliques and the contralateral external obliques. The external rotators of the same-side hip also offer some assistance in controlling unwanted internal rotation. The AOS is pictured in the figure on top of this page with its actions being demonstrated during a gait movement.

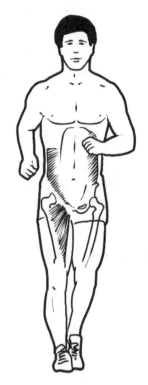

The anterior oblique subsystem.

The AOS functions through the combined actions of the hip adductors along with the contralateral obliques through the parallel alignment of their fibers. Their close proximity of attachment at the pubis allows for force transference and communication between the aponeurosis insertion of the external oblique and the origins of the pectineus and adductor longus muscles.[10] These muscles of the AOS work synergistically to stabilize the body on top of the stance leg while rotating the pelvis for the swing phase of gait. The AOS also works with the POS to help with optimal positioning of the pelvis and leg to prepare for impact from the succeeding heel strike.[12, 19] The AOS, in concert with the POS, is also instrumental in accelerating rotational movements such as the forehand swing of a tennis racquet or the right cross punch of a boxer. A cable, one-arm chest press performed in a lunge position, would be an example of an exercise to target the AOS.

The Lateral Subsystem

The *lateral subsystem* (LS) provides for stabilization and movement in the frontal plane. It is primarily composed of the hip abductor musculature: the gluteus medius, gluteus minimus, and the tensor fasciae latae that work synergistically with the lateral flexors of the trunk to the opposite side, particularly the quadratus lumborum and the internal obliques. Some assisting control from

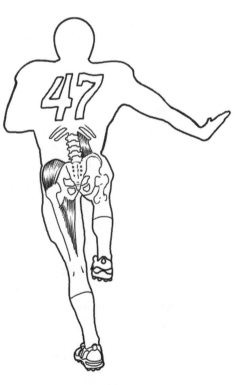

The lateral system.

the ipsilateral hip adductors is also an integrated feature of the LS. LS function is demonstrated during a sport-specific movement in the figure at the bottom of the previous page.

As the running back presses sideways off the stationary leg, the gluteus medius, minimus, and TFL activate to abduct the hip. The accompanying activation of the lateral flexors to the opposite side causes a slight lateral tilt of the pelvis to assist with the lift of the leg. With assisted control of the hip adductor complex, the LS muscles work to dynamically stabilize the pelvis and body over the shifted center of gravity. A succeeding sideways plant of the opposite leg would signal immediate activation of the opposite lateral subsystem. You can observe this similar side-to-side motion in several sports besides football, such as speed skating and tennis. The LS would be highly active during the lateral one-leg jump shown in Chapter 6, "Speed, Agility, and Power Exercises."

The Control System

The control system is the most complex system to even begin to present and attempt to understand. The complexity of the brain's physiology and countless processes is far beyond the scope of this book. Instead, I'll briefly summarize the basic functions of the central nervous system and its interactions with the various associated components of the body for both sensory input and motor control. This information is presented at a level pertinent to understanding the scientific rationale for the techniques presented in this book and for improving the bio-motor capabilities of the human body.

You can view the control, or sensorimotor, system as containing the central nervous system (CNS), peripheral nervous system, and all sensory receptors that offer information and feedback to the CNS. The figure at the bottom of this page pictures a basic overview of the control system with some of the major neural structures identified. You can find more detailed schematics in a good anatomy book if you need better reference of the numerous smaller neural structures. The thousands of sensory receptors located throughout the body, which also are critical components of the control system, are not depicted here.

We receive continual sensory information about our present environment through a number of different sensory channels. Our three primary sources for information pertaining to our environment are visual, vestibular, and through proprioception. Visual and vestibular receptors sense changes in center of gravity and play an important role in body positioning and

1. Brain
2. Cervical plexus
3. Brachial plexus
4. Musculocutaneous
5. Spinal cord
6. Radial
7. Median
8. Ulnar
9. Lumbar plexus
10. Cauda equina
11. Sacral plexus
12. Sciatic
13. Femoral
14. Tibial
15. Common peroneal

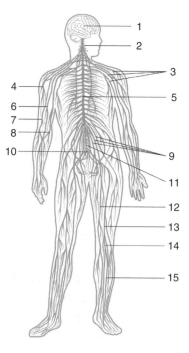

Frontal view of the sensorimotor system.

balance. Sensory receptors in the cutaneous tissues sense changes in pressure and movement of soft tissue. Mechanoreceptors located in the muscles, joints, and connective tissue give continual information and feedback on joint position, stability, and movement, muscle length, tension, and pressure from external and internal forces. All this afferent input from all three sources is processed at different levels of the CNS to generate the appropriate reflexes and motor responses.[25]

Motor responses fall into one of the three levels of motor control depending on the complexity of the information and the familiarity of the various stimuli. I'll present the primary components of each level of motor control and briefly summarize their associated functions in the following order:

* The spinal cord handles simple reflex actions.
* The lower brain organizes more complex responses.
* The cerebral cortex controls the most complicated responses and possibly stores general motor programs.

The Spinal Cord

The spinal cord is made up of two-way tracks of nerve fibers. It carries both sensory fibers and motor fibers between the periphery and brain. It allows for the continual flow of afferent information from the sensory receptors to the higher levels of control. It also contains the efferent motor fibers carrying command information from the cerebrum to the periphery organs or muscles.[25] One branch of the sensory nerves terminates in the gray matter of the spinal cord; another branch is carried to the higher levels.

This enables the spinal cord to react autonomously to certain stimuli without the need for processing of commands from a higher level of control. These reflex actions—such as quickly regaining balance after slipping on an unseen patch of ice—are critical for performance and protection of the body. Reflex actions can be improved by integrating proper training stimuli such as balance boards and stability disks. Skillfully applying unexpected forces from unpredictable angles, such as manually pushing and pulling a person while he attempts to stabilize and perform a desired movement, is another example of reflex stabilization training. This form of stabilization training might be an ideal exercise with high transference for certain athletes such as wrestlers or basketball players.

Commands are sent through the spinal cord with two types of anterior motor neurons: *alpha neurons* and *gamma neurons*. *Alpha motor neurons* are larger motor neurons that innervate the large skeletal muscles of the body. Alpha motor neurons can innervate a small amount of fibers for fine control such as for the fingers and toes. Yet, they also can innervate as many as several hundred muscle fibers in larger muscles for gross control of major joint movements. A *motor unit* is a single motor neuron and all the muscle fibers it integrates. According to the all-or-nothing theory of muscle contraction, if a signal is strong enough to activate any motor unit, all fibers of that unit will contract with maximal force. The spinal cord and brain regulate the excitation or recruitment of motor units based on sensory information and the perceived need.

Gamma motor neurons innervate small intrafusal fibers and the muscle spindles of skeletal muscle. There are two different classes of gamma motor neurons: One controls dynamic sensitivity or movement; the other controls static sensitivity or stabilization. These specialized motor neurons are constantly influenced by mechanoreceptors around the joints and appear to play a critical role in both dynamic and static stabilization of the joint.

Sensory receptors from visual, vestibular, skin, joints, connective tissue, and muscles flood the spinal cord and brain with afferent input from the environment. The receptors most involved with joint movements are often referred to as *mechanoreceptors*. Two important mechanoreceptors highly involved in muscle actions are the *muscle spindles* and *Golgi tendon organs*. Muscle spindles are located in the belly of the muscle and monitor muscle length changes or rate of change in length.

Muscle spindles are extremely sensitive to the lengthening or stretching of a muscle and have both dynamic and static stretch reflexes. When activated, they immediately signal the recruitment of motor units to create tension in a muscle, to slow down the speed of lengthening, or attempt to completely halt lengthening to protect the muscle from overstretching or any resulting damage to the joint.[25] In fact, it is this stretch-reflex of a muscle that often is a desired action that can be exploited for power movements such as jumping and throwing activities. However, "muscle pulls" are often attributed to the same stretch-reflex when an untimely and forceful muscle spindle activation takes place in a muscle that was unprepared or unconditioned for this reflex action.[35]

Golgi tendon organs (GTOs) are located in the tendon and monitor tension and its rate of change. They immediately transmit information to the CNS relating to the degrees of tension on the tendons and muscles throughout the body. When tension is suddenly increased in a specific muscle, the GTO sends an instantaneous message that can result in partial or complete inhibition and loss of contractile force in that muscle. This also appears to be a protective mechanism to preserve muscle and tendon structures. There is a dampening effect of both GTO and muscle spindle activity when exposed to the stimuli gradually or often enough that the entire system becomes conditioned to the movement. This provides a sound rationale for using gradual range and speed progressions to practice any dynamic movement before attempting it at full power.

The Lower Brain

The lower brain consists primarily of the brain stem, basal ganglia, and the cerebellum. Several descending pathways of motor control are directly or indirectly under control of the lower brain. Certain afferent sensory information is processed at this level along with efferent messages to modify or change a movement for greater efficiency.[19] The following figure pictures the brain with the different areas labeled for a visual reference.

The *brain stem* is the stalk of the brain connecting it to the spinal cord. All sensory and motor information must pass through the brain stem to reach the appropriate end organ. It contains a specialized collection of neurons that help to coordinate skeletal muscle function and modify specific control functions of the body. The brain stem also plays a significant role in maintaining balance, or equilibrium, of the body over its base of support.

The *cerebellum* assists the primary motor cortex and the basal ganglia by helping to adjust the actual movement patterns being produced to conform to the desired motor patterns established by the higher brain. The cerebellum takes relayed decisions for desired movements developed in the motor cortex and processes this with sensory information from the various receptors to decide the final movement it will attempt. It then continually monitors and compares sensory feedback and attempts to smooth out the movement, as well as eliminate inefficient responses or delays to commands. The cerebellum is always attempting to learn how to best perform a movement based on all available information. This reinforces the importance of proper input of exercise technique particularly when learning a new movement. The cerebellum also is critical for any complex movements performed in a rapid or ballistic manner such as running and jumping.[19, 25]

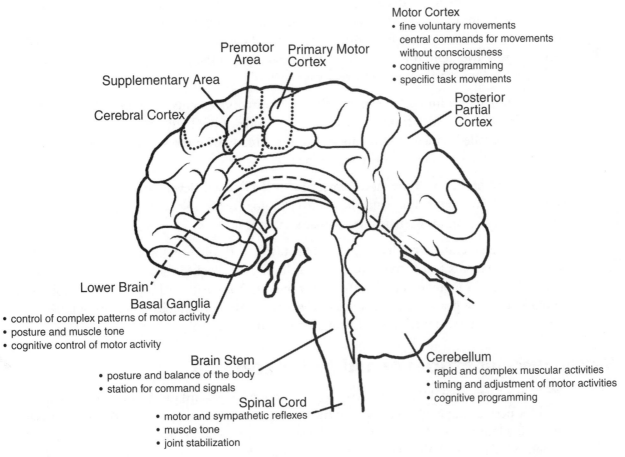

The different areas of the brain.

The *basal ganglia* also assist the higher brain with control of complex motor activities. Almost all sensory and motor nerve fibers connecting the cerebral cortex with the spinal cord pass between the basal ganglia. One of the principal responsibilities of the basal ganglia is to initiate and control repetitive and continuous movement patterns such as walking and running. Various nuclei are contained in the basal ganglia that assist the cerebral cortex with specific functions. One of these is the *caudate nucleus*, which plays an important role in cognitive control of difficult or new movements that require integration of a thought process prior to and during performance.[25]

The Cerebral Cortex

The cerebral cortex is the upper and most outer area of the brain; it consists of two hemispheres connected by the corpus callosum. The cerebral cortex controls the most complex motor patterns and is responsible for initiation of all voluntary movements as they automatically require a certain level of cognitive control. The cerebral cortex simultaneously controls the different functions and coordinates the various activities of the motor cortex with all areas of the lower brain and spinal cord. Desired motor commands along with their designed patterns are sent to the lower centers of the control system. They in turn evaluate these programs along with feedback, modify them if needed, and then pass these commands along to the active muscle system for execution. The cerebral cortex has two functional areas concerned with movement: the *motor cortex*, which consists of the primary, premotor, and supplementary areas; and the *posterior somatic sensory cortex*.[25]

The primary motor cortex controls fine voluntary movements. Its right side controls the left side of the body; its left side controls the right side of the body. It is responsible for consciously controlled skilled movements and works directly with the spinal cord through the corticospinal tract for control of reflex actions.

The premotor area of the motor cortex is involved in the development of finely skilled movement. It works together with the primary motor cortex, the basal ganglia, and the thalamus to form a system for efficient coordinated muscle activity.

The supplementary area functions synergistically with the premotor area to help with postural movements and corrections. It also is highly involved for bilateral movements of the body. This might be related to the effect that moving both arms or legs together would have on one's center of gravity. Any changes in center of gravity would challenge the supplementary area's first stated function of assisting with postural control.

Neuromuscular Efficiency and Motor Learning

The control system and the active system (neuromuscular system) can become more synchronized for performing any specific skilled motor program, such as a powerful swing of a baseball bat to hit a home run, or simply typing a document on a computer key pad. As neuromuscular efficiency is developed, this skill or task is performed with less conscious effort and with less metabolic cost. *Neuromuscular efficiency* can be described as the neuromuscular system's ability to learn, store, and recall rehearsed motor programs, complete with the required force productions and reductions, and containing the appropriate stabilization strategies and balance reflexes.

The number of possible motor programs that could be produced by the human body is an infinite combination of specific joint movements and synchronized muscle activations. To the question of the brain's capability to store all this intricate information, experts such as Schmidt have proposed the concept of *generalized motor programs*.[37] This theory proposes that general motor patterns, as opposed to specific, detailed movements, are stored in the higher levels of the brain for quick recall when needed. Then, depending on the afferent information from the various receptors, these general motor programs can be modified at the appropriate level to meet the environment. Along these lines, Chek developed a training and rehabilitation system utilizing general motor programs he termed the "Primal Pattern System™."[11]

Derived from Chek's system and logical approach to teaching exercise movements that are more transferable to life demands, I will present a slightly modified version of general motor programs. Following the research of several experts who have shown that all movement begins with movement or stabilization of the spine, I find that seven distinct general movement patterns emerge. These movements can be observed as they are being developed during the first two years of life. They are a flexion pattern; extension pattern; rotation pattern; push pattern; pull pattern; squat pattern; and finally, gait, which is further broken down into four distinct variations.

You can visualize how these motor patterns are developed in an infant as it first learns to move. Movement begins with flexion and extension of the spine while arm and leg movements lack much voluntary control. Spinal rotation and more controlled integration of the arms and legs are gradually added to roll over when desired, and for performing pulling and pushing patterns. This is needed to roll over, push up, and crawl. Eventually, more leg control develops as the infant performs assisted squat patterns to get up and down, and finally to perform beginning gait patterns to walk.

Gait begins with walking; it then varies according to need. (Lunge patterns develop to walk up steep terrains or step over obstacles. The desire or need for increased speed develops running patterns that can then be transitioned into sprinting.) These patterns are modified as our bodies change and grow. Neuromuscular efficiency of these general patterns is established and then used throughout our adult lives. The following figures picture these patterns as they might occur in our adult daily activities.

Unfortunately, while living in a modern industrialized society, lack of need to use these patterns— on a consistent basis—gradually detrains them. These movements become less efficient and more difficult to recall. Injuries, muscular imbalances, and postural deviations will further alter performance of these general movements, which leads to compensation and storing of distorted motor programs. This eventual reduction of functional movement is a reduction in the quality of life. Exercise programs that focus on integrating the proper proportion of these general movement patterns are essential to improving performance of daily activities and improving athletic abilities.

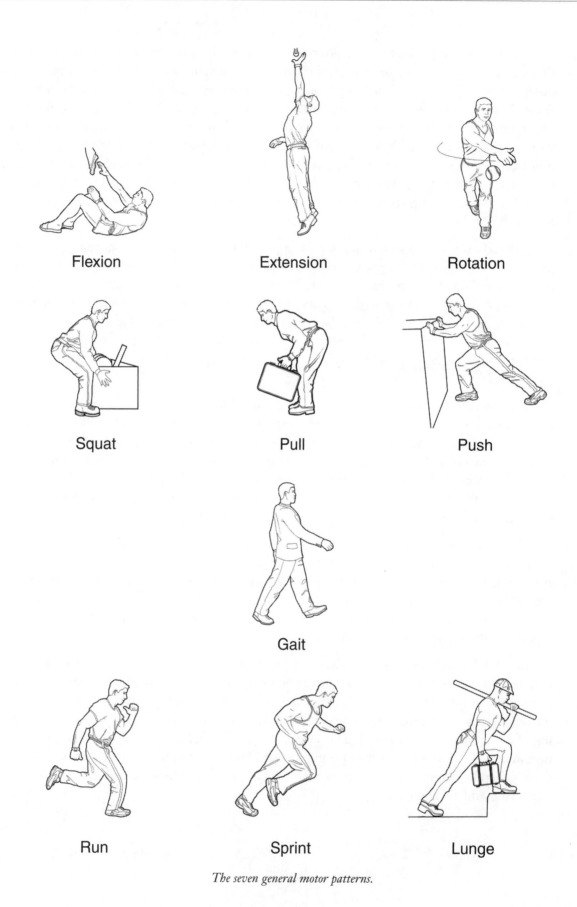

| Flexion | Extension | Rotation |

| Squat | Pull | Push |

Gait

| Run | Sprint | Lunge |

The seven general motor patterns.

Summary

The unique design of the human body allows for an infinite combination of postures and movement. The components enabling all human movement can be classified into three interdependent systems: the passive-skeletal system, the active-muscular system, and the control-sensorimotor system. The passive system is composed of the axial and appendicular skeleton, the joints, and all associated connective tissue. The active system is composed of the muscles, their tendon attachments, and their associated fascia. The active system is the link between the control and passive systems. The musculoskeletal system is the term often used to represent all the combined components of the passive and active systems, as well as their synergistic functions. The neuromuscular system is likewise the term often used to encompass the combined components and integrated functions of the control and active systems.

You can associate all individual joint movements of the passive system with specific muscles that act as either primary movers or synergists for that specific joint movement. This information is helpful for identifying the muscles responsible for certain movements. However, the body does not move in an isolated manner. The control system typically recruits muscle synergies and combines a multitude of joint movements to perform even the most basic movements needed for daily tasks. Research has identified some of these muscular subsystems that integrate to perform interdependent actions. The inner unit, or core, provides for respiratory functions while simultaneously acting as a critical local stabilization system for the spine and pelvis.

The deep longitudinal subsystem, posterior oblique subsystem, anterior oblique subsystem, and the lateral subsystems also work to provide gross spinal-pelvic stabilization. However, these outer units provide for hip and trunk and shoulder movement as well.

The control-sensorimotor system is made up of the central nervous system; the peripheral nervous system; and all sensory receptors that provide for proprioception and the gathering of all afferent information from the body and its environment. Information is processed at three different levels of the central nervous system depending on the complexity and familiarity of the stimuli. The spinal cord, lower brain, and the cerebral cortex all work together to process information, elicit appropriate reflexes, generate commands, and then learn and store this information.

Neuromuscular efficiency is the neuromuscular system's ability to learn, store, and recall rehearsed motor programs complete with the required force productions and reductions, combined with the appropriate stabilization strategies and balance reflexes.

With the infinite possible motor programs that can be created, the control system can store those generalized motor patterns used most often; these can quickly be recalled and then modified to suit the present environmental needs. It is logical that these general motor patterns would be established in the first years of our lives, then modified as our bodies and abilities continue to progress. Training that reinforces these general motor patterns should be more transferable to life demands.

Strength and Endurance, Stability and Mobility

There are several individual bio-motor abilities you can improve through training that will enhance human performance. The three most often sought after are strength, speed, and power. However, for overall health and optimal performance, it is crucial to develop all facets of human performance. All bio-motor abilities have interdependent relationships that necessitate a more balanced approach to training. It is also important to realize that individual goals will dictate which of these capabilities need to be prioritized and what unique blend of each will need to be obtained. This holds true whether training to improve athletic abilities for a specific sport or increasing general overall fitness levels for personal reasons. The following seven bio-motor abilities will be discussed here and in the following chapter:

* Strength (all specific types)
* Endurance (muscular and cardiovascular)
* Stability (includes balance)
* Mobility (static and dynamic flexibility)
* Speed (all specific types including quickness)
* Agility (coordinated use of all abilities)
* Power (combined use of strength, stability, adequate mobility, and speed)

In special cases, an elite athlete's sport might require extreme focus on a specific few abilities with an intentional neglect of others. Olympic weight lifters or shot putters, for example, who need specific types of strength, power, and stability for their events, really have little need for developing endurance. In fact, training endurance, or even learning various agility drills, might elicit neuromuscular adaptations and store confusing motor patterns that actually could decrease this particular elite athlete's peak performance. For most athletes and fitness enthusiasts, however, it is advisable to make some improvement in all abilities, at the appropriate ratios for their goals.

Strength

Of all the bio-motor abilities, I cannot think of one more important for overall fitness than strength. No other single ability can help quality of life more than increased overall strength. Strength is also a prerequisite for other abilities such as stability, speed, and power. Strength can also contribute to agility, mobility, and even muscular and cardiovascular endurance, if strength is trained in a specific manner. Despite popular belief, it is possible to train the cardiovascular-respiratory system while working in the anaerobic energy systems and developing strength.[21, 23, 27] However, no matter what other abilities are needed to accomplish the various goals of the individual, increased strength would undoubtedly also be advantageous.

Strength often is thought to be synonymous with muscle size, or hypertrophy. This misconception has detoured certain athletes and many fitness seekers, particularly women, from aggressively training for increased strength. Although gains in cross-sectional size of a muscle will add to overall maximal strength, gains in strength are related more to neurological, than structural, adaptations.[3, 16, 27] Significant gains in strength with little or no change in muscular size are very attainable with a properly designed program. Strength is in part a by-product of the control system's capability to recruit specific numbers of motor units and its integrated function with the active system for increased intermuscular and intramuscular coordination.

Intermuscular coordination is the neuromuscular system's capability to orchestrate the most efficient recruitment of agonists, synergists, stabilizers, and neutralizers for the given movement. *Intramuscular coordination*, on the other hand, is the neuromuscular system's capability to control specific motor unit and muscle fiber recruitment within an individual muscle. This process involves *number encoding*, *pattern encoding*, and *rate encoding*. Basically, number encoding is the total number of muscle fibers recruited. Pattern encoding deals more with the synchronization of the appropriate types of muscle fibers recruited, whereas rate encoding is the rate at which muscle fiber is recruited or activated.

Aside from motor unit and fiber recruitment, there are other factors that determine the overall strength of any movement, such as the lack of inhibitory responses, biomechanical factors, psychological factors, and the neuromuscular system's familiarity with the movement pattern. Genetics is definitely the most empowering, or limiting, variable for development of maximal strength. However, this does not mean that dramatic strength improvements can only be attained by an elect few. In fact, significant strength gains are most often easier to attain than are some of the other bio-motor abilities such as speed, agility, and even mobility or flexibility, since genetics also has a strong influence on these abilities as well. It has been my experience that strength gains are realized much sooner than other common training goals, such as weight loss or hypertrophy.

Specific types of strength gains are possible by utilizing different training techniques due to strength development, which is mostly related to neural adaptations in the control system. For this reason, changes in technique for certain exercises will stimulate receptor activity that alters neuromuscular adaptations, which can be beneficial for developing the desired type of strength. For example, pausing at the eccentric-isometric phase of each repetition while the muscle is lengthened is ideal for developing static-strength and starting-strength. On the other hand, working with a faster eccentric movement followed by a quick ballistic concentric movement with no pause would elicit a stretch reflex of the muscle. This would be more in line with goals of increased explosive-strength and power development. The following list explains seven basic different types of strength that can be developed with the appropriate training techniques.[38, 41]

1. **Absolute-strength** refers to the absolute maximal force output possible from a given muscle. This would take a complete override of all the inhibitory and protective mechanisms of the joint and all antagonist muscle groups. Therefore, this is more of an estimated, potential quotient of strength rather than a measurable, actual quotient. Absolute-strength would be exhibited only in extreme emergency situations.

2. **Maximal-strength** refers to the training maximal muscle force that can be expressed with a single maximal effort or repetition. Knowing this exact amount is rarely important for any training goal. Also, because safety is a concern when attempting a single-rep maximum, it can be projected through a six-rep maximum test. This usually represents about 85 percent of maximal-strength depending on the exercise and the person's individual physiological makeup.

3. **Relative-strength** is a measurement of maximal force production in a given movement divided by the mass of the individual. For example, a large male football player might display a much higher maximal-strength for a certain lift than a female gymnast. However, once body weight is considered, he might still measure at a significantly lower relative-strength level than the gymnast.

4. **Static-strength** is the muscles' ability to produce force at a specific joint angle. For our purposes, it is synonymous with stabilization, strength and most often involves a total or partial isometric contraction of the active muscles.

5. **Speed-strength** is characterized by the ability to move the body or a light load quickly. This type of strength development is ideal when the speed of movement is more important than the maximal amount of force such as when punching or kicking. Speed-strength can be further broken down into two different categories of specific strength types: starting-strength and acceleration-strength.

   * **Starting-strength** is the specific force a muscle can produce when beginning in a static, prelengthened position. Starting-strength often contributes to an athlete's quickness. Dead-lifts, as well as all the Olympic lifts, are sample exercises that require good starting-strength of the leg and hip musculature. This is because these particular lifts require the lifter to start in a deep squat position before pulling the bar from the floor.

   * **Acceleration-strength** is the capability to continue to increase force once the movement has begun. This specific type of strength typically picks up right after starting-strength and is needed more for certain movements than others. For example, a heavy dead-lift or bench press performed with a full pause at the chest would require both starting-strength and acceleration strength. Whereas, a barbell clean also needs starting-strength for the first pull from the floor, but not much acceleration-strength, as this movement can utilize the bar's momentum once it is initiated.

6. **Endurance-strength** is required when one must maintain a set amount of force over a longer period of time. This can further be displayed as *static-endurance-strength*, which is characterized by the capability to maintain a posture or joint position under load for a long period of time. It can also be expressed through *dynamic-endurance-strength*, which would then be characterized as the capability to maintain a constant level of force production for an extended period of time while in movement. An example of this is a bike-rider pedaling up a long mountain road.

7. **Explosive-strength** is the ability to produce a maximal amount of force in a minimal amount of time. A shot putter in action is a classic demonstration of explosive strength. However, some texts describe explosive-strength as most commonly displayed when utilizing the stretch reflex.[38] Adopting this view, explosive-strength is characterized by a movement that is initiated through use of the stretch reflex making it a key component for *power*.

It is important to note that increases in maximal-strength appear to transfer at some degree to all other specific types of strength within the same movement. Increases in maximal-strength will also automatically increase relative-strength, as long as the body weight remains constant. Static-strength, speed-strength, and endurance-strength also improve through maximal-strength gains, although maybe not proportionally or optimally. Explosive-strength should also improve with increases of maximal-strength particularly in similar movement patterns; for example, maximal strength gains achieved in the squat can often improve one's vertical jump. Explosive-strength and power will obviously be further improved once the stretch reflex is incorporated with the new levels of maximal-strength.

In short, for many people the type of maximal-strength gains that can be achieved through a properly designed and periodized program is often all the strengthening they need to achieve their goals. This type of program promotes proportional gains in maximal-strength throughout the body and provides enough variety of training stimuli to make some increase in all types of strength and improve all bio-motor abilities. However, elite athletes might need more specialized programs that focus primarily on specific types of strength required for their specific sport.

Endurance

Endurance is often thought to be solely an adaptation of the cardiovascular-respiratory system and associated primarily with increases of maximal oxygen consumption (*VO2 max*). This misconception has led to training protocols for endurance athletes that dramatically overlooked or completely ignored the possible benefits of strength training. The development of increased local-muscular-endurance that can be attained through resistance training is highly valuable for improved performance in endurance activities. There is always some level of strength involved in any event, as no movement on this planet is a nonresisted movement.

Local-muscular-endurance is the muscle's capability to maintain the optimal force production necessary for the movement for an extended period of time. Local-muscle-endurance derives from the development of endurance-strength. The more strength is required for the movement, the larger part endurance-strength plays in its contribution to the endurance activity. For example, research on master-level, middle-distance runners showed that a decrease in performance was attributed primarily to local muscle fatigue, which leads to compensational movement patterns and a decrease in stride-length, as opposed to cardiovascular fatigue or decreases in stride frequency.[38] In other words, the decreased performance was due more to a loss of muscular strength rather than a loss of leg speed or reduced cardiovascular endurance.

Further research comparing VO2 levels of top-endurance athletes has shown very little correlation with performance.[38] This proves that in any endurance event there are other contributing factors associated with optimal performance, apart from conditioning the cardiovascular-respiratory system and increasing VO2 max.

Conditioning programs for improved endurance should prepare the muscles for *onset of blood lactate accumulation (OBLA)*, which is the beginning of *anaerobic threshold*. This is when the anaerobic processes of ATP production for muscle contraction becomes prominently involved, which decreases aerobic power and limits endurance. Training should aim to do more than just develop lactic-acid tolerance of the local muscles; it also should strive to train the muscles to actually delay OBLA while continuing to perform optimally. Resistance training circuits and interval training can help to accomplish this. This can also be accomplished through proper endurance-strength training of the specific muscles through specialized event-training protocols.

Resistance training has been shown to obtain better gains in hemoglobin content (Petrov & Lapchenkov, 1978) and myoglobin content (Pattengale & Holloszy, 1967; Hemmingsen, 1963) than aerobic training. This is a significant fact, as increases in hemoglobin and myoglobin are critical for improved endurance.[38] This type of research confirms that the benefits of a periodized program that includes ample amounts of resistance training can help to improve the performance potential of the endurance athlete.

Endurance is not just a metabolic process, it is also a neurological one. Any movement performed for endurance will require the use of specific muscle synergies and intermuscular control. Therefore, endurance is also interdependent on specialized adaptations of the control system. Improvements of intramuscular control—such as the number, pattern, and rate encoding of muscle fiber—are also key for improved endurance.

As any endurance activity will use a predominant repetitive movement pattern, the importance of proper sensorimotor adaptation should not be overlooked. Any reflex actions needed for the event and all voluntary movement must become less cognitively controlled and more automated for greater efficiency and improved metabolic conservation. Intermuscular control, as well as intramuscular control, is crucial for optimal performance of any activity and holds true for endurance events as well. Stabilization strategies also should be more easily managed with possible backup strategies prepared, as fatigue becomes an issue. The specific environmental variables such as temperature, terrain, elements, and equipment also should be introduced to the body and the control system for adaptation and prioceptive, visual, and vestibular familiarity. All this will assist with the neuromuscular efficiency, which will increase endurance and improve performance.

It is highly probable that effective compensational patterns of movement will also need to be developed by the control system when preparing for competition in extreme endurance events such as marathons and triathlons. Even with training it is likely that all involved agonists and synergists will have different fatigue levels. Compensation strategies then will need to be activated to continue the activity or event. Compensation has definite ramifications on the programming of the neuromuscular system and places undue stress on the musculoskeletal system. However, it is a necessary action of the body for continued movement after fatigue occurs, and it often begins far before it is noticeable in performance.

Compensation and its ultimate consequences, such as the development of muscular imbalances and abnormal mechanical wear patterns of the joint, are some reasons experts have developed strong opinions on participating in long endurance events. My personal opinion is that training and competition in activities at any extreme range, whether it is long endurance events or maximal strength and power events, should not be encouraged for those simply seeking overall health and fitness. As a former competitive athlete, I realize that we do these extreme sports for a variety of personal reasons other than health, and often at our own expense.

Chapter 7, "Progressive Program Design," provides an example of how a periodized program will assist with increasing endurance-strength of the muscles and improved cardiovascular respiratory function that utilizes only moderate amounts of traditional aerobic training. Research has shown that properly designed circuit resistance-training programs can achieve approximately equivalent functional benefits for the cardiovascular-respiratory system as training programs that are based on use of traditional aerobic activities such as running.[38] This makes inclusion of additional aerobic activity more of an option for those only seeking general health and fitness.

Stability

Stability, or *stabilization*, for our purposes may be defined as the internal capability to control all desired movement or nonmovement of the body and its segments in response to the environment and changes in center of gravity. Adopting this definition means that stabilization may be a static-, dynamic-, or balance-demand, with most movements requiring a combined blend of all three. Even a simple walk around the block would require certain amounts of dynamic-stability with some contributions of static-stability, and even require minor levels of balance depending on the terrain and abilities of the person. Stability is closely related to strength, but also includes balance.

* **Static-stability demand** is characterized by the joint demonstrating complete stability through isometric muscle actions. The joint can be completely motionless or it can move in space. For example, you might observe the static stability of the spine while it is completely motionless during a dumbbell bicep flexion, or witness it during a squat movement in which the spine is again held stable, yet is allowed to move in space. Both require isometric contractions of the trunk muscles and are examples of static stability.

* **Dynamic-stability demand** is characterized by a partial stabilization of a joint while there is controlled movement in the selected planes. For example, both the hips and ankles are directly involved in median plane flexion and extension during a squat movement. However, they must be dynamically stabilized from moving into unwanted pronation or supination in the frontal plane. Dynamic-stability also is required when stabilization is needed upon quick demand to support the joints upon experiencing a sudden impact force. This can be viewed as *impact-stability demand* and is critical for any sports where jumping, quick changes of direction, catching objects, or any impact with the environment is needed.

Stabilization requires the interaction of all three of the major systems, also needed for movement. The passive-skeletal system, apart from its unique structural design and its own connective tissue, relies heavily on the assistant forces and connective tissue of the active muscular system. This system in turn receives all reflex actions and motor commands from the control-sensorimotor system. Therefore, stabilization is not an end product, but rather a continuing process during any movement that is limited by a weakness or breakdown of any one of these systems.

For example, if the control system fails to supply the proper reflex or command quickly enough, stabilization is compromised or lost. On the other hand, if the active system receives the command but lacks the muscular strength, reaction, or endurance, stabilization is again compromised or lost. In either case, you can view the passive system as the final and last resort for stabilization. Any breakdown of stabilization here results in a total or partial collapse with a high probability for deformation or injury of the joint, and possibly to other areas of the body. This provides a strong rationale for some level of stabilization and balance training in most everyone's program, despite perception of overall goals. I'll present more specific information on stabilization training in Chapter 4, "Resistance Training Technique."

Balance is an intricate part of stability and is defined as the process of maintaining one's center of gravity within the body's base of support. Balance relies predominantly on the activation of specialized reflex actions that vary from small shifting responses of the ankle or hip, to stepping strategies and associated upper-extremity movement to regain center of gravity.[25]

Balance reflexes can be divided into two major classifications: *body-righting reflexes* and *tilting-response reflexes*.[11] Although many sport and life movements, such as racing a motorcycle or simply skating around the block on a pair of roller blades, will require a specific blend of both reflex actions, most activities can be considered as a dominant demand of one or the other.

* *Body-righting reflexes* tend to dominate when standing or moving on a stable surface such as when performing a dumbbell reverse lunge off a stable step, or even a gymnast performing her routine on a balance beam.[11]
* *Tilting-response reflexes* are dominant when the supportive surface can also move beneath us, as in performing a set of squats on a wobble board or standing up in a small boat.[11]

Choosing the appropriate balance challenge is essential to training and improving the desired reflex action of the neuromuscular system. Because all balance and stabilization strategies need to be programmed, a certain volume of exposure to the stimulus is required. In other words, it must be practiced often enough for the neuromuscular system to learn the ability, and then continued it at some level for proficient recall. For example, we might never forget to ride a bike once we learn; however, this does not mean we can perform high-skill movements with the bike without continued practice. You'll find more information on training balance reflexes in Chapter 4, "Resistance Training Exercise."

Mobility

At the other end of the spectrum of joint stability is joint mobility. The integrity of every joint is dependent on both abilities, with optimal performance having the ideal ratio of stability to mobility. Some movements or activities might require greater ranges of motion; others would benefit from more stability and less available motion. Mobility is related to the joint's possible range of motion (ROM), which is difficult to determine because ROM varies under different conditions.

The type, exact direction, speed, and force of motion will alter any joint's ROM. Internal factors such as force production and reduction, inhibitory responses, muscle fatigue, inter- and intramuscular control, and arthrokinetic dysfunctions of the joint can also cause variations in ROM. Environmental factors such as temperature, presence of external loads or forces, and even the time of day also influence ROM. Simply stated, any joint can have degrees of variance at any time depending on these numerous factors.

If even the same joint on the same person can vary, one can imagine the degree of differences from person to person. The individual genetic differences of anatomical factors such as bone length, ligaments, joint capsules, tendons, muscles, and fascia can create a large divergence in estimating what a "normal" ROM should be. There are no "normal" people; only data that suggests what normal might be under identical conditions in which the data was gathered.[38] Therefore, increased joint mobility should be trained at a level based on the needs and goals of the individual; comparisons to others should be limited.

Although muscle stiffness or flexibility often is perceived as the major limiting factor to ROM, several other anatomical factors contribute to joint stiffness. A review of Chapter 1, "The Human Body: Anatomical Design and Function," will give you an idea of the components of the musculoskeletal system along with the resistance to stretching discussed for each. The following table breaks down the contribution to joint stiffness offered by various components.[6, 19]

Contribution to Joint Stiffness by Components

Structure	Resistance
Joint capsule & ligaments	47%
Muscle (fascia)	41%
Tendon	10%
Skin	2%

As the joint capsule, ligaments, and tendons are resistant to stretching; attempting to do so would be futile and permanent damage could possibly result. This basically leaves the muscle and its associated fascia, which you can target for lengthening for increased flexibility, to increase joint mobility.

Flexibility, oddly enough, is defined as all soft tissue's level of *extensibility* for allowing joint range of motion.[19] As previously mentioned, because ROM can vary depending on several factors, two basic types of flexibility are typically presented: passive and active flexibility.

* *Passive-flexibility* refers to joint ROM produced when the muscles are inactive and a force outside that joint is responsible for limb movement.
* *Active-flexibility* is when an agonist muscle is used to produce joint ROM and express the flexibility level of the agonist.

Research has shown large degrees of difference between measurements of passive ROM to active ROM; this has been termed the *flexibility deficit*. This demonstrates that an increase in passive-flexibility does not necessarily transfer to an increase in active-flexibility. Because most desired joint movements during daily activities, exercise, or during sports are of an active nature, active-flexibility is by far more important for performance than passive-flexibility. The only proposed benefit for an increased amount of passive-flexibility compared to active is the possibility of serving as a protective reserve in situations in which a sudden force takes the joint past its normal operating limit. However, research and experience suggest that the flexibility deficit correlates strongly with the incidence of soft tissue and joint damage.[38]

We know then that increased flexibility—particularly of an active type—can bring several benefits. A review of research and contemporary literature suggests that not only does an increase in active ROM reduce incidence of injury, it might also delay muscle fatigue, decrease muscle soreness, and increase performance. These are exactly the reasons we all should desire an optimal level of flexibility. So why then has stretching become so controversial?

As with any form of exercise, the problems often are with the techniques, not the exercise itself. Some experts have argued that there are no unsafe exercises, stretches, or techniques, only inappropriate prescriptions of them for the wrong person at the wrong time.[33, 38] However, many experts also agree that several traditional exercises and stretches would compromise most of the joints in such a manner that they are difficult to generally recommend. Therefore, we continually search for and suggest better alternative exercises and techniques for improving all the bio-motor abilities, including flexibility.

It is important to realize that inappropriate stretching techniques can be detrimental to joint integrity and cause permanent damage. Deformation of the ligaments, tendons, and joint capsules can be the result of overzealous efforts to increase the flexibility of a perceived tight muscle. It does not always take quick or forceful movements to cause injury, as many assume. In fact, the myotatic stretch reflex often will protect the muscle and joint when a ballistic movement is involved. Often, it is the slowly forced, passive, and prolonged stretching that results in permanent deformation and loss of joint stability.[38]

Alter states, "The outcome of any flexibility program can be made predictable and less haphazard if certain biological and biomechanical principles are understood and applied" (p. 1).[6] There are numerous stretching techniques and varying terminology in traditional and contemporary training methods. It is beyond the focus of this book to present them all and discuss the subtle differences. To simplify the different types of stretching, just remember that there are two types of flexibility. Logically then, there are two general stretching techniques: passive and active.

Passive Stretching

Passive stretching (similar to static stretching) involves the use of a force outside the joint for limb or body movement. This force can be gravity, as when simply leaning over to try to touch the toes, as demonstrated in the figure on the right. It can also be performed by using other muscles unrelated to the targeted joint to stretch with, such as pulling one arm across the body with the other arm. You can also perform a passive stretch by using another person to move the limb or body, or with the use of a machine or device. The common element of a passive stretch is that the muscles around the joint are not being activated. One of the possible advantages to passive stretching is that it can be more relaxing than active stretching, which can help with stress reduction, a major benefit by itself. Passive stretching can also provide for better adherence to a regular stretching program if it is more enjoyable.

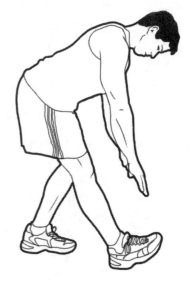

Passive stretching.

Active Stretching

Active stretching (also known as dynamic stretching) is more reliant on the voluntary activation of an agonist muscle group to stretch its reciprocal antagonist. The figure on the right shows an example of active stretching. This is accomplished by the man simply pulling one leg up off the floor as high as possible against gravity while keeping it locked at the knee and the foot dorsi-flexed. This would constitute an active stretch for the hamstrings and gastrocs. Similar movements can be done for any muscle group. Active stretching works to reprogram the neuromuscular system and decrease inhibitory action of the opposing muscles. Active stretching tends to produce more active flexibility but is specific to the rate, range, and speed of activation. Therefore, there are several different methods of performing an active stretch:

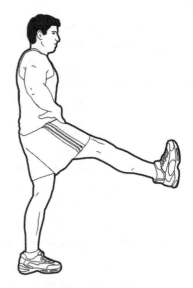

Active stretching.

* **Progressive dynamic stretching** works on the premise that the stretching antagonist muscle is sensitive to the speed and rate of stretch as well as the amount of stretch. Therefore, developing specific speed of flexibility for the required movements of the activity is also highly advisable. This method is characterized by specific imitation of the desired movement that is gradually increased in range, speed, and intensity. This is particularly a popular method of stretching just before the specific event and is often included as part of the warm-up routine for many athletes. These rehearsed movements that are gradually increased to full speed and ROM facilitate muscle synergies, as well as decrease inhibition and viscosity of tissue just before using the movement for the specific event.

  An example of this could be a martial artist practicing his kicks by progressively increasing the height, speed, and force of each kick before the competition. Another example is a sprinter warming up by starting with a slow jog, gradually increasing to a run, and then finally an all-out sprint coming out of the blocks. In Chapter 6, "Speed, Agility, and Power Exercises," I recommend the use of a similar progressive dynamic stretching technique. You can accomplish this by simply beginning each movement pattern or drill at half-speed, and then gradually increasing the speed, range of motion, and power of the movements so that by the fourth or fifth repetition you are at full intensity.

* **Contract-contract stretching** is characterized by a preceding voluntary contraction of a muscle followed by a quick voluntary contraction of the opposing muscle. This technique is designed to decrease antagonist muscle inhibition and increase activation of the agonist needed for improved range of active flexibility. The figure on the right demonstrates a common contract-contract technique for improving active amounts of hip flexion and lengthening on the hamstring musculature. This technique can be used for targeting improved active ROM for practically any joint.

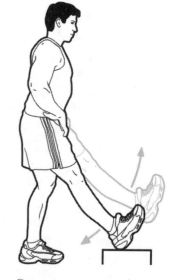

Contract-contract stretching.

Passive-Active Combinations

Passive-active combinations use combined stretching techniques, which you can also do through either contract-relax or relax-contract techniques. Contract-relax requires a partner who assists with a voluntary contraction of the opposing muscle to be stretched, followed by a relaxation of that muscle combined with an immediate assisted passive stretch. This is designed to decrease inhibitory response and is a basic version of Proprioceptive Neuromuscular Facilitation (PNF) stretching. The relax-contract technique begins with a relaxed passive stretch that is held at maximum ROM, followed by an active attempt to further ROM. If successful, the next passive stretch begins with the new ROM, followed again by another active attempt for increased ROM.

PNF is not just a stretching technique … it is rather an entire clinical approach to flexibility, neuromuscular programming, and joint stabilization. The scope of this system is beyond the focus of this book; however, I have adopted several PNF concepts—not only for the aforementioned stretching techniques, but also for integration into some of the strength and stability exercises. Those familiar with the total PNF system will recognize the valuable influence it has made on the philosophies and techniques presented herein.

Summary

There are seven basic bio-motor abilities you can strive to improve for increased levels of fitness or in order to achieve optimal performance. Although strength, speed, and power may be deemed the most important, it is also important to develop all bio-motor abilities at the proportional amounts based on individual needs and goals. No other single ability could be considered any more important for overall fitness than strength. Many of the other abilities expressed by the body such as stability, speed, power, and even endurance are reliant on certain levels of strength for improvements.

There are several specific types of strength that can be trained in order to obtain specific goals. Depending on the demand of the sport or activity, the need for increased maximal-strength, relative-strength, static-strength, speed-strength, endurance-strength, or explosive-strength will vary. There are exercise techniques and programs that can be utilized to elicit these specific strength adaptations, many of which are presented in this book.

Endurance is the body's ability to maintain performance of a certain activity and repeated motor patterns for prolonged periods of time. Endurance is often wrongly thought to be only a metabolic adaptation of improved VO2 max and cardiovascular-respiratory performance. Research confirms that local-muscular-endurance and neurological adaptations, as well as specific strength improvements, can all contribute immensely to overall endurance.

Stability is not an end result, but rather a continual process of the integrated functions of the control, active, and passive systems of the body. It may be defined as the internal capability to control all desired movement or nonmovement of the body and its segments in response to the environment and changes in center of gravity. This means stability can be a static- or dynamic-demand and includes balance strategies and reflexes. There are two basic types of balance reflexes: body-righting and tilting-response reflexes. You can use specific training techniques to target these different reflex actions as needed for individual goals.

Mobility, most commonly referred to as flexibility, is another important bio-motor ability that can improve or impede performance. There are several features of the musculoskeletal system that determine how much flexibility, or range of motion (ROM), is available at any given joint. These structural limits should be understood before attempting any stretching program or activity, as inappropriate stretching habits can cause permanent deformation of connective tissue and decrease joint integrity. There are both passive and active stretching techniques that can safely and efficiently increase relative passive and active ROM. As most life and sports movements depend more on active than passive ROM, active stretching should be included in any comprehensive training program.

Speed, Agility, and Power

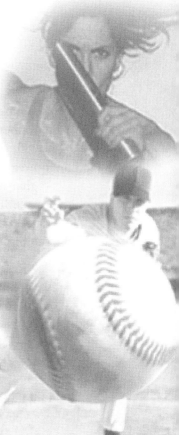

Speed, agility, and power are arguably the most critical attributes to an athlete's success in numerous sports. They are the remaining bio-motor abilities involved in optimal human performance and are the focus of this chapter.

All bio-motor abilities are a product of the combined functions and interactions of the body's passive, active, and control systems, and all have interdependent relationships. The key for developing increased speed, agility, and power lies in first developing a prior blend of improvements in specific types of strength, stability, mobility, and endurance. This is precisely the reason those abilities were presented first before discussing speed, agility, and power.

Traditional belief has been that one could develop each bio-motor ability separately, and then summate them for the desired end result or for optimal performance. However, based on recent scientific findings and practical experiences, several experts now consider these approaches antiquated.[38] Because the neuromuscular system is much like a programmable computer, it needs the proper input on how each of the specific improved abilities needs to be combined for use in the final program. In other words, the fact that an athlete might have improved his or her strength in the gym, speed on the track, flexibility, balance, agility, and power is no guarantee that he or she will perform any better in his or her particular sport. The athlete must now combine these improved abilities through sport-specific practice in the precise motor programs needed for his or her sport. Otherwise, these improved abilities lay in wait as nothing more than potential.

This is not to say that you can't train in progressive blocks by focusing more effort and time on developing one or two abilities per cycle. In fact, this is what progressive training and periodization do. For example, in the early stages of development I highly recommended that you spend most of your efforts improving strength, endurance, stability, and mobility before beginning high-speed, agility, or power training. This establishes a strong, stable, and safe fitness foundation prior to beginning speed, agility, and more ballistic types of training. Performance can only be built as high as the base can support. The following figure shows a basic diagram depicting this training philosophy of the important roles and working relationships among all the bio-motor abilities.

Speed

Speed is one of the most difficult bio-motor abilities to improve. Its interdependent relationships with mobility, stability, and endurance are often overlooked, and its reliance on strength is also often underestimated. Depending on the way you need to exhibit speed, you will need to develop a specific mix of maximal-strength, relative-strength, explosive-strength, speed-strength, and endurance-strength. This speed and strength relationship is important to remember, as many coaches and athletes have come to believe that improving speed is next to impossible. This perception often results from failures in running programs that did not spend adequate time improving strength or utilized only traditional training techniques.

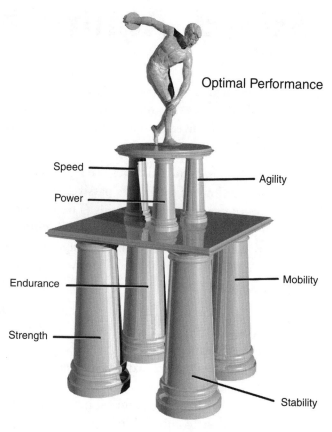

Bio-motor abilities for optimal performance.

There is no doubt that genetic factors set certain physiological limitations for maximal speed, as they do for every other bio-motor ability. However, they do not prevent most people from making significant improvements on current levels of speed if they are willing to learn the necessary processes and are dedicated to performing the required work.

Research on muscle physiology shows that all muscles are composed of a mixture of different fibers divided into two basic types: *fast-twitch* and *slow-twitch*. The fast-twitch fibers are the key for speed, as they can produce higher levels and faster rates of force and provide for greater power output.[23] Therefore, people born with a higher ratio of fast-twitch fibers will have a higher potential for maximal speed, whereas people with a greater genetic distribution of slow-twitch fibers would typically be more adept at endurance activities. However, further research has pointed out that there actually is a continuum of several different types of muscle fibers ranging from the type I slow-oxidative fiber to the type IIb fast-glycolic fiber.

Research has identified at least nine different muscle fiber types that demonstrate the capabilities to adapt to different training stimuli.[21] This continuum of muscle fiber types and their correlation to performance in different energy systems is discussed in Chapter 7, "Progressive Program Design." Research suggests that most of these fibers can shift their ability to perform slightly different functions in response to training.[21] This means that different subtypes of IIa slow-twitch oxidative-glycolic fibers that are designed mostly for muscular endurance can learn to perform better for speed and power demands if trained properly. This range of adaptability holds some promise for increased speed but is still limited, as it is unlikely that any type I slow-twitch oxidative fibers can ever be trained to perform like fast-twitch glycolic fibers.

Genetic structures of the control system also have been cited as a limiting barrier for maximal speed. Elite sprinters appear to have more organized central nervous systems. Their bodies often contain reticular and spinal cord systems capable of transmitting much higher frequencies of discharges than the average person.[38] In other words, reflexes and commands from all three levels of control are sent at faster and more frequent rates. How much of this is adaptive to their training and participation in competitive events versus how much of it is simply genetics is inconclusive. However, we do know that the control system is programmable and sensitive to training, so improvements in speed as related to adaptations of the control system are possible. It is also important to note that these adaptations of the control system take longer and are less noticeable than the structural changes of the active-muscular system.[21, 25, 38]

Speed and Strength Relationships

Through proper training of specific types of strength you can attain both physiological and neural adaptations to improve your potential for maximal speed. Any increases in maximal-strength, as previously discussed, appear to offer some carry-over benefits to all types of strength increase. Maximal-strength increases are due more to neurological adaptations and the improved use of larger amounts of fast-twitch muscle fibers. These adaptations are also conducive to increasing maximal speed. Therefore, it is logical to assume that gains in maximal-strength (particularly of the core and trunk muscles—shoulder flexors and extensors, and the hip flexors and extensors), should potentially help to increase speed.

It is logical to assume that this would also have a higher carryover if this strength was developed using more generalized motor patterns such as free-weight squats, lunges, and standing pushing and pulling exercises. However, it is important to remember that with resistance training, it is the amount of load that recruits more fast-twitch fibers, not the speed of movement. You will compromise maximal-strength gains and development of fast-twitch fibers if you spend too much time attempting to move lighter weight loads with faster tempos.

Improvements in both components of speed-strength, starting-strength, and acceleration-strength are obvious ways to help develop increased speed. This specific type of strength training does focus more on the speed of movement rather than the amount of resistance; however, you cannot do this effectively with the heavy free-weights used for maximal-strength development. There are other training tools and techniques more suited for developing speed-strength such as using weighted sleds, parachutes, or even elastic bands or straps for partner-resisted and partner-assisted running exercises. Stadium stair running, running in sand, or sprinting in a pool are other common methods of attempting to develop increased speed-strength. Emphasis of training priorities for developing the different components of speed-strength depends on the present abilities of the person and the demand of the specific activity. The development of starting-strength is important for any speed goal, where athletes must begin in stationary positions and move within more limited spaces. Tennis players, soccer goalies, and short-distance sprinters are examples of athletes that would need to focus more on improving starting-strength than other athletes. The first few steps of speed are often termed as one's *quickness*.[9] The need for quickness is prevalent in many sports and often requires both starting-strength and acceleration-strength depending on whether the athlete begins from a stationary position or is already in motion.

Athletes involved in sports with more constant motion, who need sudden bursts of speed to cover longer distances, would want to focus more on acceleration-strength. *Acceleration* is most simply defined as the process of increasing velocity, or speed. Rate of acceleration is often more important than maximal speed for these individuals to catch a ball or overtake an opponent. Studies on elite athletes who have comparable maximal speed have demonstrated high degrees of variances in acceleration.[23] These differences can be traced directly to the varying levels of acceleration-strength and is particularly important for athletes competing in field and longer court sports such as football and soccer or hockey and basketball.

Speed-strength is also directionally specific. Some people need to improve lateral speed and quickness, whereas others need more straight-ahead speed. Backward speed and diagonal speed might also be needed for optimal performance in certain activities. Many athletes need to generate speed-strength in a variety of directions that can change at any given moment. In any case, these specific movement patterns must be learned, modified, and rehearsed before they can be stored and recalled for immediate use. Simply increasing the tempos of resistance training exercises and learning to run faster down a track will not meet the specific speed-strength demands for most athletes. Specific sports training drills and actual practice of the sport itself are the most transferable methods of developing speed-strength for athletes.

Relative-strength increases are also very important for gaining greater speed for many people; this is a matter of simple physics. The amount of body weight compared to strength will directly affect overall speed more than strength itself. In fact, a reduction of body fat coupled with a moderate strength increase could do more for achieving greater speed than a high degree of strength gain coupled with no weight loss, depending on the resultant relative-strength ratios. A diet and overall exercise program designed to reduce body fat and maintain muscle often is imperative in these situations.

When you need speed for quick and powerful actions while on the move, explosive-strength is vital to develop. Explosive-strength is derived from use of the stored elastic energy produced from fast, eccentric, or lengthening actions of the muscle. This elastic energy is coupled with a fast, voluntary concentric action of the muscle to propel the body or limb in the desired movement. Explosive-strength is needed for quick changes of direction and for more powerful movements such as jumping or throwing. Sports such as volleyball, basketball, football, and baseball all have frequent demands for explosive-strength.

Endurance-strength is important to develop when you need to maintain maximal, or close to maximal, speeds for longer periods of time. A long run-back in football, or a break-away run in rugby or soccer are examples of endurance-speed derived mostly from present established levels of endurance-strength. Endurance-speed is an entire continuum representing a ratio of needed speed to endurance, with endurance-strength being the most prominent where more speed is desired. Long-distance running or swimming events are related more to straight endurance and require less endurance-strength. This relationship triangle of strength, speed, and endurance again demonstrates the interdependence of various biomotor abilities and the need of individuals to develop their own unique mix to perform at optimal levels for their specific goals.

Speed and Other Bio-Motor Relationships

Joint mobility is also an extremely important factor for improving speed. The range and speed of allowed active joint motion are dependent on the various connective tissues and all antagonist muscles to the specific movements. If for any reason antagonist muscle tissues feel a need to inhibit, or attempt to halt, a movement, not only will you compromise speed, but injury is also likely. It is important to remember that these tissues must be prepared not only for the range of movement, but for the speed and force of movement as well. For this reason, regular active stretching done with a progressive dynamic technique is extremely helpful for performing high-speed movements. Inclusion of this type of flexibility training as part of a warm-up before practice or participation in high-speed activities is highly recommended. This not only prepares antagonist muscle tissue to allow for high-speed movement, but also prepares the entire neuromuscular system by recalling and rehearsing specific motor patterns before activating them at full speed.

Joint stability, particularly dynamic-stability, is also a necessity for high-speed training or activities. With higher speeds comes eventual higher impact. I'm using the term "eventual" because studies of ground forces show there is significantly less overall impact on the feet at a full sprint than during a moderate run or jog.[25] This is because of the body's established forward momentum when moving at higher speeds and the reduced actual amount of contact being made with the ground. However, eventually the movement must end, often with a sudden stop that will require large amounts of joint stability to absorb this force and protect the joint.

When discussing hand speed as opposed to leg speed, the same increased need for joint dynamic-stability can be observed as speed of motion increases. An example is a boxer's need for increased dynamic-stability from the wrist all the way down to the ankle, to absorb the greater impacts associated with faster, more powerful punches. A pitcher's increased need for dynamic-stability to decelerate the arm after throwing his fast ball is another example of the stability-to-speed relationship that is present even for more upper-body-dominated movements.

Speed and Running Mechanics

Mechanical analysis of a running gait, as presented in the following figures, is similar to that of a walking gait, although the movement does vary. Gait is often broken down into three phases: swing, stance, and propulsion.[12] However, some authors use different terminology when analyzing a running gait, such as the recovery, support, and drive phases, respectively.[23]

The swing, or recovery, phase is signaled by the impact with the ground, which is a heel-strike during running or a toe strike when sprinting. The less time is spent on the ground, the faster the movement will be and, typically, the less associated impact forces due to the increased horizontal momentum. Elastic and kinetic energies are stored from the eccentric loading of the leg during heel-strike that will be used for the subsequent propulsion phase. The swing phase is characterized by a pulling action of the leg and a rotation or torque of the pelvis, which begins the use of the stored elastic energy and the transition into the subsequent propulsion phase. The stance, or support, phase is characterized by the momentary single-leg position that occurs during transition of swing into propulsion. During sprinting this brief stabilization of the body over one foot is almost nonexistant. The propulsion or drive phase is signaled by the heel lift and push off of the ground. Remaining stored energy is released and combined with the forward momentum of the body into a powerful action that propels the body up and forward, creating the stride length between the next impact of the contralateral foot and the beginning of the next stance phase.

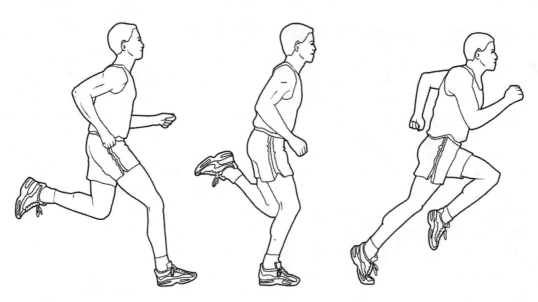

Swing, or recovery, phase.   *Stance, or support, phase.*   *Propulsion, or drive, phase.*

Any lack of mobility or breakdown in stability, or reduction of speed-strength or endurance-strength in this sequence of events will not only affect the speed but compromise mechanical efficiency, increase metabolic cost, and induce muscular compensation, which can lead to injury and increased mechanical wear of the joints. For the neuromuscular system to produce efficient running or sprinting movements, balanced muscular strength, stability, and flexibility need to be present and maintained to avoid creating faulty motor engrams and possible detrimental running mechanics. For this reason, beginning runners should consider running for shorter distances and stopping well before experiencing fatigue to establish efficient running technique. You can do additional conditioning with a variety of other aerobic activities if needed, until the running distance is gradually increased to the desired amount.

You can assess two measurements of running technique for possible improvements: the stride-length and stride-frequency. Either one can be measured fairly easily and recorded for future comparisons. It is important to realize that an increase in either one at the expense of overall technique typically will slow overall speed. Other authors have made similar observations when working with people who were incorrectly taught to overemphasize stride-length. The effort to mechanically produce the exaggerated stride-length resulted in such a decrease in stride-frequency that they experienced diminished levels of performance and an overall reduction in speed.[25] Many experts assert that with use of form running exercises and regular sprinting training, the ratio of stride-length to stride-frequency will naturally be worked out by the neuromuscular system for the best functioning of the person's own anatomy. Research has demonstrated a significant degree of variance between stride-length and strength-frequency even when comparing athletes with almost identical maximal speeds.[38]

Agility

Performance is reliant on much more than a person's genetic potential for maximal speed. The constant stopping, starting, and change of direction involved with most sports makes it unnecessary for most athletes to ever express maximal speed. It takes Olympic-level sprinters 60 yards to reach top speed. This distance is rarely covered in any one burst during any sport other than track and field. This fact also leaves recreational athletes or fitness enthusiasts with little reason to worry about actual maximal speed, as it is probably unnecessary to achieve their goals.

As speed begins to be manipulated for the sudden stops, starts, and changes of direction for the given sport or activity, coordination of quickness, specific strength needs, stability strategies, and balance must be also managed. This coordination ability is known as *agility*. Agility is difficult to define as it is the culmination of nearly all other bio-motor abilities a person processes.[23] I define it as the outward display of the individual's level of *neuromuscular efficiency*. This means agility is the capability of the neuromuscular system to efficiently store, recall, modify, combine, and execute several motor programs simultaneously while concurrently processing visual, vestibular, and proprioceptive information to continue to refine the actual movements.

Whereas improvements in maximal speed are often difficult to achieve and might have limited benefits for overall performance, agility is more often the contrary. Proficient agility requires the neuromuscular coordination of flexibility, dynamic stability, balance, specific strength development, speed, quickness, power, and even endurance depending on the duration of the activity. Therefore, agility training integrates and implements improvements in any one of these abilities, which can show immediate results in performance depending on the characteristics of the activity. In other words, individual gains in strength, flexibility, speed, or power will not always show improvements in performance until the neuromuscular system has had experience integrating the specific improvement into more complex motor patterns through agility training or activity-specific practice.

Agility and Coordination

Neuromuscular coordination is a process, as the related systems for improved intermuscular and intramuscular control, increased reflex activity, and faster responses to feedback from afferent receptor information all take repeated exposure to the stimuli in order to improve. Neuromuscular coordination for increased agility is refined through three basic stages, as identified by Verstegen and Marcello,[23] and coincides with the Fitts's model of motor learning.[19, 37]

* **General-coordination or cognitive-control:** This stage is characterized by the need for cognitive, or conscious, control of voluntary movement. The person must think through the movement as he or she is performing it, relying heavily on visual and auditory input as proprioception information is too new and unfamiliar at this stage.

* **Special-coordination or associated-control:** At this stage, the person has become more comfortable and begins to feel the proper movements. The person has less reliance on visual and auditory information and more use of proprioception. The individual installs stabilization and balance strategies and utilizes feedback information to refine the skill and discard undesired motion.

* **Specific-coordination or autonomous-control:** This stage is the highest level of motor learning. It is characterized by the performance of the skill through stored motor programs with no conscious thought. The neuromuscular system carries on with automatic reflex actions and response commands to all environmental variables; the movement pattern is free of all superfluous motion.

Agility and Speed Training

Armed with this information, it becomes clear how a logical progression of a training program should flow. Time is always a precious commodity, and energy is a finite resource. Therefore, it is logical to spend the most time on something that will offer the most results based on individual needs and overall goals. For example, too much emphasis on increasing maximal speed might be the time and energy better spent on agility training for most athletes and fitness enthusiasts. This book presents exercises for improving both speed and agility in Chapter 6, "Speed, Agility, and Power Exercises."

I chose to present speed and agility exercises that do not need any ergonomic devices or additional resistance tools. As previously mentioned, bands, parachutes, and stadium stairs are popular for increasing running power and development of maximal speed; however, they are not readily available to everyone. Cones, ladders, and hurdles are also valuable tools for agility training but are not presented as needed tools in this book for the same reason. The assistance of a coach or trainer for directional commands and immediate feedback on performance is also a valuable and highly recommended addition for speed and agility training. However, this book aims to provide the reader—whether he is a trainer, coach, athlete, or fitness enthusiast—with exercises that can be done safely without the use of devices, special tools, or reliance on another party.

Power

Athletic power is a key for overall performance in many sports. Activities that require any quick and explosive movements (such as jumping and throwing), or those that require the swinging implements such as bats, clubs, or racquets, rely on power for optimal success. Power is a mathematical formula typically expressed as Force × Velocity. Velocity can be further broken down into Time ÷ Distance. Basically, this means that power is the combination of one's strength times his speed of movement. However, there are other prerequisites for increasing the potential for power that are often overlooked. Joint stability, mobility, and even endurance can also be important ingredients for optimal power. Proper programming of the neuromuscular system and the ability to exploit the stretch-reflex are also necessities in power production.

To express power, you must overcome Newton's Law of Inertia, which states that a body at rest or in uniform motion will stay at rest or uniform motion until acted upon by another force.[23, 25] This means that to quickly move an object at rest or already in motion, its inertia plus any additional momentum must be overcome with a quick production of force. Think of how often additional power would be beneficial—not only for athletic movements, but also certain daily activities. Bounding up a flight of stairs, jumping and swinging the body over an obstacle, or simply rising quickly from a chair are examples of powerful actions that can be advantageous in certain life situations.

Physical therapist, author, and well-known expert on power training Dr. Donald Chu says, "Power should be viewed as the icing on the cake and not the cake itself" (p. 84).[23] This practical analogy implies that there are several ingredients needed for preparation of the cake before applying the power icing. You can compare strength and speed to the primary ingredients of flour and water that make up the cake, while dynamic stability, appropriate joint mobility, and endurance can be the sugar and flavoring additives. To expand further on this analogy, consider the time it would take the neuromuscular system to combine and bake these ingredients before applying the icing. Much like agility, power is toward the end of a process that progressively developed several other bio-motor abilities.

At least 8 to 12 weeks of pretraining are recommended by Dr. Chu before beginning an aggressive power-training program,[18] with 21 weeks cited in the program progression example provided in Chapter 7. The actual time period depends on the person's present needs, abilities, and overall goals.

It is also possible that for general health and fitness goals, aggressive power training phases are not necessary at all. Whenever power of movement is increased, a subsequent amount of increased stress and strain is placed on the involved soft tissues. Stress is described as "the amount of force applied to and absorbed by the body." *Strain* is described as "the ability of the body to absorb these forces and recover from them" (p. 84).[23] Certain amounts of stress and strain are inherent in all types of training as mentioned previously, but often can be adapted to if experienced in moderate doses and progressed slowly. In fact, it is the adaptation to stress that provides the desired effects. Therefore, neither stress nor strain are automatically considered detrimental unless the stress occurs at levels or rates that cause an overstrain on the tissues, resulting in compensation, undesired deformation of tissue, or injury.

Power Prerequisites

Several capabilities should be developed before progressing to an aggressive power training program. This section provides a comparative checklist to help determine a person's readiness for power training.

* **Core control and trunk strength:** As I discussed in Chapter 1, "The Human Body: Anatomical Design and Function," these two terms are not synonymous. Core control relates to the strength development and ability to voluntarily and autonomously activate the inner unit when desired or needed. This local stabilization system of the spine and pelvis is a protection mechanism, and is also highly involved in production of any powerful movement of the body. Also, powerful movements often involve ballistic flexion, extension, or rotational movements of the spine that the outer trunk muscles will need to accelerate and decelerate for optimal power and protection of the musculoskeletal system.

* **Joint integrity:** You need appropriate levels and ratios of stability and mobility of involved joints for safe and efficient production and reduction of power. Joints too stable or stiff will slow movement and reduce power, whereas joints too mobile or unstable can inhibit power and are more prone to deformation of soft tissues and injury. Dynamic-stability, improved balance reflexes, and active-flexibility are all important prerequisites to power training.

* **Endurance-strength and endurance-speed:** These are more helpful for power training than most realize. Even though the quick production of force and velocity is an ability that results from the anaerobic processes of ATP and energy production, recovery from any activity is highly dependent on the aerobic system. For improved recovery between sets and the increased ability for prolonged training sessions, prior conditioning of endurance is beneficial.

* **Agility and power training:** These go hand in hand for most training goals, as both require similar prerequisites. Power should be trained with agility by applying the *SAID*

Principle, which states that the neuromuscular system has "Specific Adaptations to the Imposed Demands." This means that improved power should be integrated into specific agility and sport-specific training to achieve optimal performance. Throwing a medicine ball, for example, only ensures improvements at throwing medicine balls, which to my knowledge is not a sport or athletic event yet. The improved power derived from such exercises eventually must be applied to the specific movements involved in the activity.

Plyometrics and the Myotatic Stretch Reflex

Plyometrics is a training system highly popular in power training programs. This effective form of power enhancement is characterized by the use of the myotatic stretch-reflex and utilizes stored elastic energy for creating powerful movements. Plyometric training has been around for some time; its roots are in Eastern Europe and it is believed to have been formalized as a discrete training system known as "shock training" in Russia during the early 1960s by scientist Dr. Yuri Verkhoshansky.[38] World interest in plyometrics, also known as *jump training*, did not develop until the early 1970s, when Eastern Bloc countries were producing superior athletes in events such as track and field, gymnastics, and weight lifting.

The term "plyometric training" comes from the naturally occurring plyometric actions of a muscle during movements such as running and jumping. The natural stretch-shortening cycle of muscle contraction has a naturally occurring reflex termed the *myotatic stretch-reflex*, which can produce more power when used with an appropriate voluntary contraction of the muscle. The mechanisms of the stretch-reflex are highly detailed and involve the integrated functions of the control, muscular, and skeletal systems. The stretch-reflex is believed to be a designed function of the neuromuscular system for joint protection, as well as for mechanical efficiency. Following is a brief summary of this process for better understanding of the science behind plyometric training.

As a muscle is eccentrically loaded during what is termed the *amortization phase*—particularly when done with high velocity, or speed—elastic energy is immediately stored in the tendon and serial elastic components of the muscle for the subsequent concentric action. The mechanical delay period between eccentric and concentric muscle contraction is known as the *coupling time* and is a far shorter period than the time it would take to activate any voluntary contraction through cognitive control. Immediately following the eccentric stretch is the forceful concentric contraction known as the *summation phase*. Combining this stretch-reflex muscle contraction with the appropriate voluntary movement produces a much more powerful movement than that of a voluntary muscle contraction on its own.

A vertical jump test is an easy demonstration to compare additional power offered by the stretch reflex. For the first attempt, simply begin by positioning the body at the bottom of a squat position. Starting from a dead stop, explode upward and reach as far as possible, making sure to mark the highest point. Then attempt the vertical jump, beginning in a standing position, and perform a quick drop into the squat position, followed by an immediate explosive jump. Compare the two heights; the latter movement should have produced a significantly higher jump. The difference in height is known as the *power deficit*. The smaller the deficit, the more possible power gains from plyometric training, as the neuromuscular system has not yet learned to exploit the stretch-reflex to its full potential.

However, practical experience has shown that some elite athletes can produce high power from stationary positions as well as when proceeded with an eccentric movement. This might make this practical comparison less accurate for predicting plyometric value, as these individuals can often still make significant progress through use of this training system.

Power Training

Chapter 6, "Speed, Agility, and Power Exercises," provides instruction for several plyometric and medicine ball exercises aimed at developing added power. This small sampling of the myriad of exercise options represents the easiest to learn—yet the most efficient in terms of power development. I selected exercises that begin in a variety of postures and develop power movements in all three planes of motion. Other than a medicine ball (preferably a power ball that offers a moderate degree of bounce), no other devices, tools, or training partners are needed.

As with the speed and agility exercises, there is optional equipment such as boxes and barriers that can be used for plyometric training and a wide selection of medicine balls and rebounders that could be used for upper-body power training. However, I did not want to rely on too many tools for the exercise selection and programming used in this book. I also did not include the various exercises that need help of a partner or a trainer. As a professional trainer myself, I know the added benefit of working with a skilled coach or trainer, but also realize that this might not be a training option for everyone. Besides the exercises for developing power presented in Chapter 6, there are also programs provided in Chapter 7 that demonstrate how to implement power exercises into a periodized program. These programs present a method for developing the required prerequisites of power, then gradually progress into programs containing more plyometric and aggressive power training routines.

Summary

High levels of speed, agility, and power are all attributes most often needed for optimal performance of many athletes. These important bio-motor abilities would also be advantageous qualities to possess for any fitness enthusiast or active person. However, prior development of strength, endurance, stability, and mobility provides the body with the necessary base needed to launch any aggressive training programs designed to enhance athletic performance.

Speed is often thought to be the most difficult bio-motor ability to improve. Though there are genetic limitations to any other ability, speed is interdependent with strength, so it *can* be increased to a certain degree with proper training methods. Development of maximal-strength in similar movement patterns may offer some benefits, but specific speed-strength training offers more transferable adaptations for overall speed development. Starting-speed and acceleration-speed are directly associated to established levels of starting-strength and acceleration-strength. Developing these specific types of strength will help improve your quickness, which is typically more important than overall speed for optimal performance in most sports.

Agility is another highly important bio-motor ability needed for optimal performance; it depends on the integrated functions of the passive, active, and control systems. Agility combines all other bio-motor abilities and is the expression of one's neuromuscular efficiency. It can, therefore, be described as the ability of the neuromuscular system to efficiently store, recall, modify, combine, and execute several motor programs simultaneously while concurrently processing visual, vestibular, and proprioceptive information to continue to refine the actual movements. Coordination is a vital part of agility with all movements being classified into three different levels of control. Cognitive-control characterizes those movements that require the greatest levels of voluntary neuromuscular control. Associated- and autonomous-controls are progressed levels of coordination that characterize movements accomplished through more feel and less conscious thought.

Power is often a key for athletic success in many sports, particularly those that depend on the abilities to jump, throw, or swing implements. Power is often represented with a mathematical formula of Force × Velocity, which translates to your level of strength and the speed at which you can generate it. However, power is actually the end product of a process involving prior development of other abilities as well. Increased levels of core control, trunk strength, dynamic-stability, active-flexibility, and even endurance can also be important ingredients for optimal power. Neuromuscular programming for more efficient intermuscular and intramuscular coordination and learning to exploit the myotatic stretch-reflex are also critical elements in maximal power production.

Resistance Training Technique

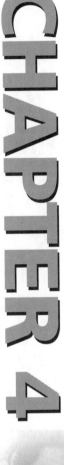

For any exercise to be as efficient and safe as possible, the specific technique is the most critical variable. I deliberately chose the word "variable," because opinions and philosophies on exercise technique are abundant in the sports and fitness fields. This is most apparent when it comes to resistance training. Several elements comprise any training technique, and it is the way you perceive these elements that will dictate the overall performance of an exercise.

Many traditional resistance exercise techniques were developed in the gym through trial and error methods. Trainers and athletes often approached them with predetermined goals, such as the desire to gain more muscle mass or move heavier weight loads. Many fitness trainers gave little regard to the study of functional anatomy, actual biomechanics, or even simple physics in the early development years of resistance training.[33]

Some of the resultant techniques, which are still in use today, are lacking in-depth analysis of resisted human movement. The human body is more than a collection of bones and muscles; it is composed of highly integrated and interdependent systems. The active-muscular system responds to reflex actions and commands from the control-sensorimotor system that is constantly processing sensory input and feedback relating to the body and its environment, to better control all movements of the passive-skeletal system. Therefore, you should consider all exercises relative to their benefits and risks for the entire body, as opposed to looking only at the individual muscles the exercise targets.

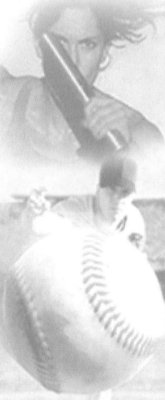

Through research of the joint structure and designed functions of the human body, and with consideration for biomechanics and the laws of physics, modified and new exercise techniques are now available. The resistance training exercises in this book incorporate this updated information and are instructed with the most efficient and safest techniques available to our knowledge. This chapter provides the background information for the scientific rationale for the elements involved in exercise technique. This in no way covers all of the underlying anatomical, biomechanical, and physiological factors that numerous experts and authors have researched over the years in order to develop the training techniques presented herein.

There are seven identifiable elements that comprise technique and should be considered when performing any resistance training exercise.[2, 3, 5]

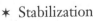
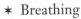

* The overall goals
* Exercise motion
* Alignment
* Positioning
* Stabilization
* Breathing
* Tempo

In the following sections, I will offer details on how these interdependent elements work so that you can fully appreciate how they are then combined to provide a foundation and framework for any resistance training exercise. By learning to identify these critical elements of exercise technique, I hope you will be able to apply them to the numerous other available exercises that may not be presented in this book.

The Overall Goals

Determining the overall goals probably is the most important element of technique, and should be done before selecting the exercise itself.[1, 2, 31] These overall goals will dictate several training variables and will affect all other elements of technique. Therefore, different goals will inevitably produce different training techniques. To best accomplish overall goals, you will often need to make modifications in the movement, alignment, positioning, stabilization strategies, breathing, and tempo. However, it is important that all modifications be consistent with biomechanical factors and kept within the anatomical limits of the body. When determining the overall goals for any exercise, consider the following factors:

* General training goals
* Specific goals and needs of the individual
* Neurological and musculoskeletal demands

General Training Goals

Motivational speakers such as Steven Covey suggest that we always "begin with the end in mind" when planning for any desired outcome; this holds true for any resistance training exercise. Before beginning, we should know why we are choosing this particular exercise and performing it in a specific manner. The general goals should be clear to the persons performing the exercise and anyone involved with instructing, training, or coaching them. Examples of general goals include increased maximal-strength, greater muscular endurance, better stability and balance, increase of speed and power, or improvements of any combination of the bio-motor abilities.

The general goals for performing an exercise and any modified technique also should be consistent with present program design factors. For example, certain elements of technique such as positioning options, stabilization demands, and tempo can often be changed according to the energy system and the muscle fiber types you target during specific training phases of a mesocycle.

Specific Goals and Needs of the Individual

You also should consider the individual person's needs or specific goals before selecting exercises and techniques. Rehabilitative concerns, muscular imbalances, and postural deviations are examples of individual needs that can affect certain elements of technique such as ROM and body positioning options. Specific and personal goals can also affect the way an exercise can be performed. For example, the desire for increased muscle mass may lead to positioning options that include more external support and use of slower tempos for increased time under tension. Often, there is a conflict between someone's needs and goals; some exercise techniques can address both. For example, a person might have a strong personal goal of increasing the size and shape of the biceps, and yet have an impending need for lower-back and pelvic stability. You can address both of these seemingly unrelated goals by applying a specific technique for a traditional exercise. For example, the following figure demonstrates a woman performing a dumbbell bicep flexion in a lunge position, using a piston movement with a moderate tempo, as an option for combining these needs and goals.[5]

The asymmetrical stance and slight forward lean of the lunge position increases static strength demands for the hip, pelvis, and trunk while the piston action of the arms continually shifts the loads and the body's center of gravity. This requires additional stabilization and slight balance reflex actions from the hip, pelvic, trunk, and inner core musculature. All of this would be advantageous training stimulus for someone in need of increased lower-back and pelvic stability.

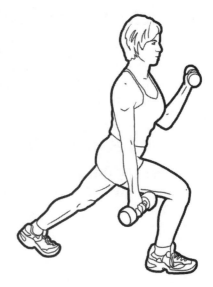

Optional technique for specific goals.

However, the movement being performed is still an almost isolated flexion of the elbow, targeting the biceps and done at moderate speed with perhaps only a slightly reduced load that would still be appropriate for hypertrophy goals. Obviously, there are other exercises and techniques that also would need to be in the program to better accomplish these specific goals and needs. However, applying these types of techniques that can address a need while still pursuing a goal is highly valuable for continued adherence to the program.

The Neurological and Musculoskeletal Considerations

Resistance training has traditionally focused on the desired training effects for the muscles, but rarely has recognized the potentially beneficial neurological adaptations. Because every exercise is simply a rehearsed set of motor patterns, perhaps you should think more about the benefits of the movement itself. Although few resistance training exercise movements will be exactly duplicated in a sport or life movement, many provide similar general movements or train the body in specific positions that transfer to movements and postures that are usable outside the gym.

You should consider that the amount of proprioceptive activity and the specific neurological demands of an exercise are factors to be considered for overall goal determination. For some people's specific goals and needs, it is not important that every exercise in the program is high in proprioception and neurological challenge. However, for others with more sports and performance goals in mind, these factors become more important to maximize the results of their resistance training efforts. Exercises and techniques that offer a more proprioceptively enriched environment with higher levels of neurological challenge are a higher priority for these people.[11, 19]

There are also several musculoskeletal considerations to consider as part of the overall goal. It is important to remember that in addition to any benefits, in any exercise there is also stress applied to joints and inherent physical risks to the body. You should compare possible risks to all joints and their connective tissues to the perceived benefits for the exercise. You should also consider the capability of all primary movers, assistors, neutralizers, and stabilizers to perform their synergistic functions. Limitations of any joint or muscle in the kinetic chain will affect the function and movement requirements for all other joints and develop compensation and faulty neuromuscular control.[19] Often, small modifications in positioning, or slight changes in stability demand or the range of motion, will reduce the risks without significantly decreasing the benefits.

The Exercise Motion

The exercise motion itself is probably the element that varies the most in resistance training. This type of motion dictates the use of all individual joints, the recruitment of all involved muscles, and the specific motor patterns to be learned. Therefore, the type, path, range, and specificity of motion are all critical factors of exercise technique.

Type and Path of Motion

Physical therapist and biomechanics expert Tom Purvis sees the exercise motion as the first of his six steps for performing any resistance training exercise. He states that the motion probably is his most important step and is closely related to, if not totally dependent on, the overall training goals.[31, 33]

There are basically only four types of movement that can be attributed to any object, or four pathways through which an object may travel.[26] Therefore, human movement can be specified according to the following classifications:

* Rotary motion
* Linear or translatory motion
* Curvilinear motion
* General plane motion

Rotatory motion is the movement of an object or segment around a fixed axis in a curved path.[26] For the purposes of this book, any isolated joint movement where the joint is stabilized is considered a rotatory movement. This type of uniplanar motion is most often prescribed when trying to isolate individual muscles for bodybuilding goals. However, exercises performed in fixed rotatory paths such as most bicep and tricep exercises, or knee flexion and extension machine movements can place high stress on the isolated joint and increase mechanical wear. These movements also have very little carry-over to any life or sport movements.

This is one reason I teach slight accessory movements of related joints to the one we are targeting. For example, if targeting the biceps is an important goal, you should perform an accompanying slight flexion of the shoulder in concert with the flexion of the elbow. This not only reduces stress and wear at the elbow, it also trains the shoulder to better support and work with the elbow during loaded flexion patterns, which is closer to how these two joints work together in real-life movements. Also, the flexion of the shoulder encourages scapular depression and thoracic extension for better stabilization of posture. At times it might be necessary or desirable to train muscles and joints in a totally isolated rotatory fashion. However, after you isolate them, you should always integrate them into the more transferable movement patterns you will use in life.[11, 15]

Linear or *translatory motion* is the movement of an object or segment in a fixed path.[26] No individual joint moves in a linear motion without the co-commitment of another joint.[10] Even then, the human body does not produce true linear movement very efficiently. Therefore, performing exercises in a fixed linear path, such as when training on a smith machine, leg press sleds, or hack squat machines tends to produce translatory forces across the joints, resulting in additional shear of joint surfaces.

When choosing to move in linear pathways, it will always take a compound movement of two or more joints and is best performed with free weights or cables that do not restrict the path of movement. These modalities will accommodate the small shifts of the joints as they work within their natural *curvilinear* structure.

Curvilinear motion is the combination of rotatory and linear motion.[26] Technically, because no joint of the body is constructed completely rounded or flat, all human joint motion also is curvilinear. As the joint rotates over or glides along bony articular surfaces, slight shifts in the axis result in a curvilinear movement of the distal end of the segment. However, because the shifts are so slight, individual joint movements are still most often classified and considered rotatory movements.[26]

General plane motion is described as the rotatory or curvilinear movement of a segment around an axis that is also in movement in the same plane.[26] Most of our traditional exercises have been taught and performed in one general plane of motion, whether they are single-joint isolated movements or multiple-joint compound movements. An exercise example of a general plane movement could be a squat. If viewing it from the side, you might see the bar move in an almost straight linear path, which can be considered a linear movement. However, the individual rotatory actions of the hip, knee, and ankle all take place relatively in the median plane. Therefore, it is also considered a general plane motion.

These general plane movements dominate our training. This could be partly because we have viewed human movement in a restricted, three-plane system. More diverse exercises that promote movement patterns traveling through all three planes have begun to emerge in contemporary training philosophies as an attempt to train more functional movements. However, there are obvious safety concerns of moving loads through different planes because each change of direction would take the effort of an entirely different set of muscles and require different sets of joint motions. What is an ideal load for certain muscles and joints might be inappropriate for those forced to take over as the resistance switches paths of movement. Therefore, these multiple plane exercises should always be done with weight loads selected for the weakest link of the chain in mind.

Although not an official classification of motion, several authors refer to these "multiple plane motions" when describing their views on movement relative to daily activities, sports movements, or when designing exercise techniques.[9, 11, 23] Occasional use of multiplanar movements may be helpful for dynamic stability, balance, agility, and perhaps even for producing power from a variety of positions and in multiple directions.

Range of Motion

One of the most debated issues in resistance training concerns range of motion. Traditionally fitness professionals believed that training with a full range of motion (ROM) is what brings about the most benefits and is what is preferred for joint health and performance. Upon investigation, I found that much of the debate is related to the combatant's view of what "full" actually means.

For many, ROM is viewed by how far the bar or weight traveled, where others look more at the joint for determining ROM.[30] From a technical standpoint, "full" means complete, such as when there is no more left, or no more room available. This is hard to determine with a joint because often more ROM is available as long as you are willing to incur damage and possible injury to connective tissues. Therefore, to better understand ROM, let's discuss the factors that influence ROM such as musculoskeletal limitations, internal and external forces, the sensorimotor system, and the goal.

As described in Chapter 1, "The Human Body: Anatomical Design and Function," the musculoskeletal system is the combined components and functions of the passive-skeletal system and the active-muscular system. Three major components comprise the passive system— the bones, joints, and connective tissue.[10] Any movement of the human body is dependent on the interaction of these components.[1,2] First, let's consider the bones and how their design may impose limitations to ROM.

Once analyzed, it is apparent that the bones are designed in a purposeful manner for a number of individual and combined functions. The bones provide for the protection and support, as well as supply the lever systems necessary for movement of the body. Each bone's unique construction allows for certain amounts of movement in specific directions while further restricting the movement in other directions. For example, the shallow concave shape of the *gleniod fossa* (shoulder socket) allows for a great amount of motion for the attached humerus. It is by far the most mobile joint on the human body, giving us an extreme amount of possible movement patterns in all directions.

However, more mobility also means less stability, and upon further analysis of the shoulder joint you will see restrictions set by the shape of the bones. For example, once internally rotated, the humerus is limited in abduction before it comes close enough in contact with the acromion process to impinge certain musculature and the bursa. Therefore, exercises that potentially force the shoulder into this internally rotated and abducted position, such as upright rows and steep decline barbell chest presses, might not be the best choice for accomplishing a given goal.

When analyzing anatomical bony barriers, it also becomes apparent that the ROM of one joint often is dependent on the movement of another. For example, once the shoulder is externally rotated it appears that there is now possible 180 degrees of abduction available. However, further investigation reveals that at least 30 degrees of that movement actually have to come from the coordinated movement of the scapula; otherwise, the shoulder joint would have to move beyond its designed limits.

The scapula has a large, flat surface designed to rotate smoothly over the posterior rib cage in all directions in rhythm with the shoulder joint. This scapular-humeral rhythm provides for extra motion in all directions and reduces stress of the shoulder joint. However, if the curvature of the thoracic spine is too kyphotic, or rounded, scapular-thoracic rhythm is disrupted, which alters scapular-humeral rhythm. In other words, shoulder ROM is also dependent on spinal positioning and the ability to stabilize proper posture. This means that people with poor posture will lack safe ROM of the shoulder joint, particularly with overhead movements. Therefore, any resistance training exercise that involves shoulder motion also should provide instructions for spinal positioning and scapular movement as a part of the technique.

Study of bones surfaces, as well as their shapes, can also help us to make better choices in regards to range of motion. The location and thickness of articular cartilage on bone surfaces gives us information on where and how far the motion is designed to travel. For example, studying articular cartilage of the hip shows that the joint prefers loaded flexion and extension of the femur while in a standing position, such as when squatting, to the similar action performed in a seated position, such as when using a leg press.[33] Excessive ROM will also take certain joints into positions where little or no articular cartilage is present and also greatly reduce the amount of joint surface contact. This will quickly place undue stress on the joint and increase mechanical wear. Articular cartilage is critical for joint health and is not easily replaced, so excessive wear of joint surfaces should always be avoided.

Another limitation to joint ROM imposed by the musculoskeletal system is from the various other connective tissues. A joint of the body is the meeting place of any two bones. Bones are held together by fibrous tissue known as *ligaments.* The elasticity of ligaments is low and they most definitely are not designed to stretch. Any significant stretching of a ligament beyond its intended design, and short of tearing, will often cause permanent deformation and reduce its capability to stabilize the joint.[6]

Tendons of a joint complex attach the muscle to the bone and, like ligaments, are very resistant to lengthening. Any lengthening in the muscle tendon unit typically comes from the muscle itself, as tendons are also prone to deformation and tearing if exposed to a significant stretching force. In fact, the stretch reflex used to generate additional power for any movement is thought to be a protective mechanism of the muscle tendon unit to keep it from being stretched too far. Since this stretch reflex is used for producing increased levels of power, any damage to a tendon will reduce overall power and make it more prone to repetitive injury.[6, 23]

Another component of the joint that affects ROM is the joint capsule. Although the capsule has more elasticity than ligaments or tendons, they also have plastic characteristics that help to stabilize the joint and to transfer forces from a working muscle to the adjacent bone. This means they also are at risk for damage with ROM outside their designed limits. Because most of the capsule, ligaments, and tendon characteristics are predetermined by their structures, research suggests that almost half of the flexibility or movement ability at any joint is determined by these structures and one's genetics. Even of the 41 percent of joint ROM attributed to muscles and their associated fascia, these tissues also have predetermined genetic allowances for ROM that vary from person to person. In other words, some people are just born more flexible than others, and anytime a joint ROM is forced past one's genetic limits, you can expect only damage and decreased performance.

Despite this fact, muscles are still the most perceived limit to ROM. Often, if a range of movement is limited, the first conclusion many make is that the opposing muscle must be excessively tight or inflexible. This perception then leads us to believe that stretching the opposing muscle would be the answer to increasing joint ROM.

It has been discovered that the lack of ROM in a joint might be often due more to agonist weakness or inhibition than to antagonist tightness. In fact, the tightness of the antagonist is often a direct result of the inhibition of the agonist. This condition could be the result of a previous injury, surgery, neural interferences, or adaptations to chronic exposure to poor body positioning or postures. In such cases, clinical facilitation and reactivation of the agonist muscles may be required to restore optimal ROM.

Probably the most significant way in which muscles can limit ROM is through active insufficiency. I defined this in Chapter 1 as the diminished capacity of a muscle to produce active tension once shortened or lengthened too far.[3, 26, 30] Therefore, if targeting a certain muscle is at all part of the goal, keep the ROM to a level at which the muscle can maintain active tension and produce force. This is particularly true for muscles that cross over two or more joints, as they are more prone for active insufficiency when they are either shortened or lengthened over both joints simultaneously.

An example of this is the gastrocs during a bent-knee calf extension. The gastrocs are preshortened by the bent positioning of the knee, so as the heel is pulled up, it shortens from its attachment at the heel and quickly becomes actively insufficient. This leaves the soleus to lift most of the load, which is fine if targeting the soleus was the original goal. Active insufficiency can also occur by extreme lengthening. For example, if the gastrocs are stretched too far, such as when performing a standing calf exercise and dropping the heels down as far as possible, active insufficiency occurs, once again leaving the soleus to lift the load with little assistance. Therefore, I do not recommend this ROM in a standing calf extension if targeting the gastrocs is the goal.

Another fact concerning muscles and ROM is that they simply fatigue during every repetition performed in any resistance training exercise. This clearly shows us that we must consider ROM a variable in exercise technique rather than a constant. For all other elements of technique to be maintained—particularly alignment, positioning, and stabilization—you must allow the motion to decrease slightly as the muscle fatigues. ROM is the most prominent concern of technique when I see lifters compensating by using additional muscle actions, changing positioning, losing stabilization, increasing tempo, and forgetting totally about proper breathing mechanics. This results in a loss of the original overall goal in order to attempt the completion of a predesignated ROM.

The study of the concurrent force systems that occur with any joint motion reveals another possible limit to joint ROM. The pull of a muscle is always a resultant pull of numerous muscle fibers, all in slightly divergent directions. This means that while a muscle appears to be contracting in one general direction, it is also applying other forces to the joint.

The muscle will always produce a rotational force in one direction in order to rotate the joint and move the bone, while generating a translatory force at the joint in a divergent direction. This translatory force either compresses the joint, distracts the joint, or creates a shear force across the joint, and typically can change during a large ROM. Study of these translatory forces shows that they increase proportionally to the amount of resistance and generated muscle force. It is also a fact that certain ranges of motions will increase compression, cause distraction, or increase the amount of shear at the joint. The range of motion of certain exercises in this book has been modified for these reasons as well.

ROM of any exercise is not totally determined by the musculoskeletal system; in fact, ROM may even be more dependent on the control-sensorimotor system. This system includes the mechanisms in which all sensory information is obtained, processed, and then utilized to generate motor commands that are then transferred back through the spinal cord to the peripheral nervous system. These impulses excite and inhibit the proper concert of muscle actions to produce the desired ROM.[25] The amount of muscle activation the nerves can control varies at different ROMs, particularly when confronted with higher levels of resistance. Simply stated, it is often more difficult to maintain muscle tension on a target muscle when using larger ranges of motion and using heavier loads as other muscles must assist more.

The loss of tension in the target muscles requires compensational efforts of the synergists for assistance to maintain ROM and might not be in line with the overall training goals. In such cases, it may be better to reduce ROM rather than continue with motor patterns that do not efficiently train the target muscles. ROM can always be increased once more neurological control of the muscles has been progressed.

In fact, every exercise is a movement first and should be trained as pure movement before loading. The body has been referred to by Chek as a "biocellular computer with a programmable sensorimotor system" (p. 46).[11] He also has often quoted Schmidt, whose research hypothesizes that it takes more than 300 repetitions of a movement before the sensorimotor system can efficiently store this pattern in memory for quick recall.[37]

Therefore, we can see the logic of always beginning a new exercise with light-weight loads and reasonable ROM until the neuromuscular efficiency is developed for that movement and it can progress in intensity and possibly ROM. Once the movement pattern has been efficiently stored and learned, we can slightly, and purposefully, modify ROM during certain training phases with little worry of developing poor engrams or faulty movement patterns.

Specific training goals can sometimes dictate a certain ROM and even be inconsistent with the overall goal. For example, the overall goal of a person may be to improve overall strength and joint integrity. However, he might also have a specific goal of bench-pressing a certain amount of weight in a competitive meet. If the person uses the ROM dictated by the sport of competitive power-lifting for his lifting technique, he must touch the chest with the bar for it to be considered a successful attempt. Depending on the person's individual anatomical limits, this ROM might be detrimental to the joint capsule and connective tissues of the shoulder, compromising his overall goals for a specific temporary goal. You can use the same analogy concerning the ROM of the competitive full squat compared to the compromised position of the lumbar spine, as it is often forced into loaded flexion because of individual anatomical limitations. In these situations, it is crucial to reevaluate the importance of the specific personal goal as compared to the compromise of the overall goals, and decide if the benefit is really worth the risk.

Specificity of Motion

All exercises are simply movements made up of a collection of stored motor patterns.[29] For this reason, many experts focus more on the motion than they do on the involved muscles and joints themselves. Many experts, such as a famous strength coach and author Vern Gambetta, often say we should be training overall movements, not just muscles. This is not to say that we should completely ignore the beneficial effects for the involved muscles, but rather consider the value of the pure movement itself. The "SAID Principle" (which stands for "Specific Adaptations to the Imposed Demands") states that our bodies will always attempt to adapt to every aspect of a physiological, neurological, and even psychological stress encountered. Therefore, we should make note if the motion itself is of any direct or indirect benefit for our training goals.

Although all the specifics of any given exercise movement will not completely transfer to life or sport movements, experts believe there is value in *general motor pattern compatibility*. This concept, as presented in Chapter 1, states that the brain cannot efficiently store and recall all the possible movement patterns that could be produced in a person's lifetime.[37] As a result, the brain stores general movement patterns that can easily be recalled and then modified when needed. Adapting from Chek,[11] these general movement patterns can be classified into seven distinct motions that are developed early in life and then continually used and modified. These movements can be broken down into flexing, extending, rotating, pushing, pulling, squatting, and gait. Gait can be altered depending to the specific demand of the movement and relative to the environment. Gait is classified into four different modifications: walking, running, sprinting, and lunging. These general movements were illustrated in Chapter 1 as the "seven general movement patterns."

Exercises that reinforce these general movement patterns are often considered "functional" movements. However, because the movement is interdependent with the goal, any movement (in my view) can be "functional" if applied to the proper goal. Often you must use isolated, nontransferable movements to strengthen weak links before progressing to a compound or "functional" movement. At times, you must also perform seemingly unrelated movements that might provide an indirect route toward an end goal. In all these cases, if the exercise is accomplishing its specific goal, then it can be considered functional.

Alignment

Forces can be broken down to their core physics and classified into either a pushing or pulling force. Alignment is the correct matching of these basic two forces. Muscle physiology demonstrates that a muscle tendon unit can actively only contract, or shorten. This action is classified as a pulling force.[26] Therefore, all muscles can only pull; none can push. The only way to lengthen a muscle is through the active shortening of the antagonistic muscles or from the application of an outside force. For the purposes of this book, alignment is defined as matching the pull of the muscles in opposition to the pull or push of the resistance.[1, 2, 4]

The muscles pull on the bones, which in turn act as a series of levers that can either pull objects toward us or, through the proper combination of pulls, create a pushing force that moves objects away from us.[10] For achieving optimal alignment, it is important to understand that all pushes the body creates are actually the combined pull of two or more muscle groups. For example, the positioning of the hands on a barbell chest press affects the alignment of forces. This pressing movement is a pull of the pectorals and deltoids to horizontally adduct the humerus, combined with the pull of the triceps to extend the elbow. Therefore, before choosing hand positioning, we must determine which set of pulls are desired to be aligned against and which resulting muscles will be targeted.

Placing the hands at shoulder width or narrower aligns the resistance directly over or inside the shoulder, meaning there is a limited amount of resistance for the adduction of the shoulder, as well as limited work of the pectorals and deltoids. There is, however, a high amount of resistance aligned in opposition to the extension of the elbow and a resultant amount of work for the triceps. If a tricep press is the goal, the shoulder-width hand positioning is appropriate, but I suggest keeping the elbows in and working in the median plane to reduce stress on the wrists, which would occur when pressing in the horizontal plane. When targeting the chest, a wider grip that aligns the hands over the elbows with the arm forming a 90-degree angle is suggested. This aligns the push of the weight load in better opposition to the pull of the chest and deltoids.

You can make similar observations for any pushing exercise, such as foot placement on a leg press machine. A lower position will challenge the pull of the quads more and stress the knee joints at a greater degree, whereas a slightly higher foot position will create an increased challenge for the hip extensors and direct more of the stress toward the hip joints. However, if choosing different positions and alignments for targeting certain muscles, understand the consequences as well as the perceived benefits. For example, a foot position placed too low in an attempt to recruit more quadriceps results in an increased amount of compressive and shearing forces at the knees, particularly if the heels come off the platform. Conversely, you also could place the feet too high in an attempt to better target the glutes. This often will force a flattening or flexion of the lumbar spine, which applies high levels of compressive forces on the lumbar vertebral disks, particularly if the tailbone is lifted off the pad at the bottom position. This can be extremely damaging over time, especially when high loads are used.

As with any of the six other elements of technique, alignment is always interdependent on the goals. Keep in mind that because alignment deals with force application, the integrity of the musculoskeletal system should not be compromised for the pursuit of any goal. Upon further investigation it is clear that to maintain a balance of efficiency and safety, alignment options are usually limited to small adjustments to slightly skew force application. You can do this for a desired effect or to get a variation of intermuscular and intramuscular recruitment patterns. An example of this is to purposefully position the body at an angle slightly out of alignment to the pull of the resistance before beginning a cable, standing, one-arm lat row. The body is positioned so that the pull of the cable pulls the arm across the body at the down position. This applies an increased rotational force to the pelvis and spine. The resulting effect is increased stabilization demand on the entire posterior-oblique-subsystem.

Numerous examples are available once alignment is fully comprehended. However, to do this you must match all other elements of technique appropriately. Alignment is not only interdependent with the goals, but obviously with the desired motion as well. In fact, to align the opposing forces, you must first know the type of motion needed to accomplish the goals. Alignment is also reliant on positioning and has little value without stabilization. Even breathing techniques and the tempo of an exercise can shift alignment during an exercise, making it less efficient.

Positioning

Positioning is another general term often used to convey different meanings. In the format for this book, positioning is the precise manner we choose to set the body and place all of its segments before and during any resisted exercise. Positioning, as with any other element of technique, is dependent on the goal. Positioning is also determined according to the desired motion and goes hand in hand with alignment.[1, 2, 3] To know how to position the body, you must first know all relative specifics concerning the alignment of internal and external forces. Positioning is reliant on stabilization and balance for proper maintenance and can even be affected by breathing and tempo.

Positioning of the Spine

During any resistance training exercise, it is important to consider the positioning of every joint of the body from the ground up, with the most critical segments typically being the spine and pelvis. The spine is the primary component of the axial skeleton and, along with the attached rib cage and pelvis, provides us with the main support structure of the body. The spine also houses the spinal cord, which is a part of the central nervous system and is the key communication line from our brain to the rest of the body, including vital organs and glands.[32]

The unique design and structure of the spinal column not only provide support, they provide for mobility in all three planes of movement. This combined role of providing stability while allowing mobility makes the spine an important factor not only in resistance training exercises, but in the execution of any dynamic sports or life movement where both roles are required simultaneously. The exact positioning and movements of the spine that are strengthened during a resistance training program will determine the positions and movements in which it will perform best during sports and life activities.

Optimal Posture

Other than exercises for targeting the outer-trunk musculature and movements designed specifically for improving spinal motion, all other resistance training exercises will position the spine in what I will simply call *optimal posture*.[19] When the spine is positioned in optimal posture, it appears to straighten; but in fact, barring any dysfunctions or muscular imbalances, it still has its optimal curvatures in place. Only a slight straightening effect of the thoracic region is noticeable in optimal posture when compared to natural posture. This is in response to the slightly increased retraction of the scapula and associated extension of the thoracic region, to better stabilize the spine from flexing under load. The following figure shows the spine positioned in optimal posture as compared to its various movements.

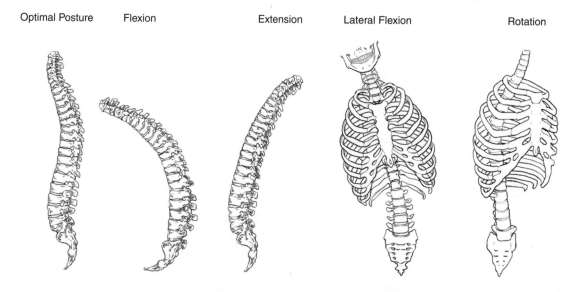

Optimal Posture   Flexion   Extension   Lateral Flexion   Rotation

Optimal posture and movement.

Optimal posture provides for optimum structural and functional efficiency of the entire kinetic chain.[19] It promotes optimum length-tension and optimum force, coupling relationships of all the muscles originating from the torso, pelvis, hip, and shoulder girdle. This directly affects the strength and function of all these associated muscles, which in turn affects the function and synergistic actions of all other muscles and joint movements of the body. The farther the spine travels from optimal posture in any direction, the less mobility it has in all other directions of movement and the less stable it becomes.

As the spine moves, length-tension relationships between agonists and antagonists change, which further reduces their ability to stabilize or produce force. All spinal movement also decreases vertebral space and increases disk compression. This is not to say that all movement or disk compression is bad; in fact, vertebral disks rely on compression forces from spinal movement for obtaining nutrients. However, it is important to remember that spinal movement, particularly passive movement under load or at high speeds, always results in proportionally or even exponentially increased degrees of compressive forces on these disks. This can dramatically increase the risk of injury and should be evaluated compared to the relative benefits of the exercise and in relation to all training goals.

Spinal positioning must be also accompanied by pelvic positioning. Other than slight sacroilliac (S.I.) joint movement, there is no pelvic movement possible without accompanying movement of the spine. An anterior tilt of the pelvis is coupled with lumbar extension; posterior pelvic tilt is a result of lumbar flexion. Associated hip flexion and extension, respectively, also accompany these described pelvic tilts.

For these reasons, when positioning the spine for any exercise, also consider the pelvic positioning. Proper positioning is important not only in the gym, but also during life movements. The following two figures demonstrate high-risk and reduced-risk positioning choices both in and out of the gym. Spinal positioning is equally important in sports, but is much more complex, as the spine is typically required to dynamically move in and out of optimum posture. I will present the proper execution of numerous speed, agility, and power movements in Chapter 6, "Speed, Agility, and Power Exercises."

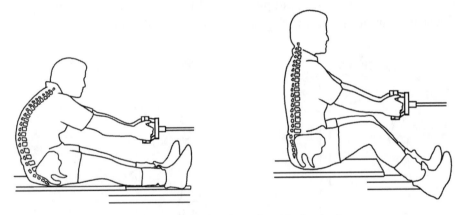

High and reduced risks of spinal positioning in the gym.

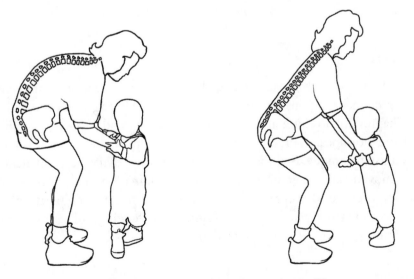

High and reduced risks of spinal positioning in life.

Positioning Options for Different Goals

At times, you can make changes of positioning options, as long as they do not significantly disturb the alignment of forces, are still efficient for performing the desired motion, do not compromise any part of the musculoskeletal system, and can be efficiently stabilized. These optional positioning choices are often used to accomplish different specific goals in a training phase. For example, a one-arm lat row can be performed in a variety of positions for different training effects, as seen in the following figures.

You can perform this exercise in a symmetrical stance with the arm braced against an inclined bench, or any stable object at the appropriate height. This position takes advantage of an outside anchor for added stabilization; this might be appropriate for a beginner who needs additional support, or it can be ideal for the advanced lifter working with maximal loads during a strength phase of his or her training cycle. You can also perform a similar exercise in an asymmetrical, or lunge, position, with no external support. This position will require a much higher demand of the glutes and quads of the forward leg for support, and a higher stabilization demand of the core and trunk muscles. This might be a positioning option selected for increased trunk and pelvic stability, or for simply loading the glutes at an increased level and targeting the entire posterior-oblique-subsystem.

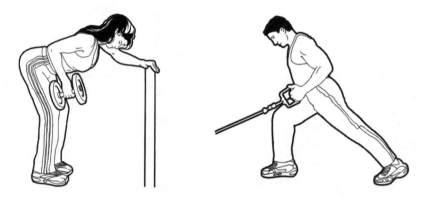

Braced symmetrical positioning (left) and unbraced asymmetrical positioning (right).

Stabilization

Stabilization is the internal ability to control all desired movement or nonmovement of the body and its segments in response to the environment and changes in center of gravity. As I discussed in Chapter 2, "Strength and Endurance, Stability and Mobility," stabilization is one of the seven basic bio-motor abilities we can target for improvement, but it is also an important element of exercise technique. Stabilization can be a static-, dynamic-, or balance-demand. Most dynamic movements are going to need some combination of all of these types of stabilization. Training exercises that offer no external support and include positions that require increased demands of stability and balance are more challenging, offer more proprioception, and are more transferable to life and sports demands.

Types of Stability

There are two basic types of stability: *static* and *dynamic*. Static-stability is characterized by the ability to hold a joint position against resistance. This is related to one's static-strength, often called isometric strength. Static-stability can be observed while the joints are motionless, such as the pelvis and spine might be held in optimal posture during a cable lat row. Static stability may be also required while the stabilized joints are in motion in space. Visualize how the pelvis and spine are in motion during a squat or lunge movement, yet still remain stabilized in optimal posture.

Dynamic stability is characterized by the type of stability a joint must exhibit while articulating to control the range and path of motion in the selected plane. For example, you might need to rotate the spine for a given exercise, but it must still be dynamically stabilized to avoid extreme degrees of rotation and prevent undesired amounts of flexion or extension. Dynamic stability is also necessary to stabilize joints upon impact, such as the ankle and hip during the heel strike in gait. This type of dynamic stability can be referred to as *impact-stability*.

Balance Demands

Balance is definitely an intricate part of stability. Balance is defined as the process of maintaining one's center of gravity within the body's base of support.[25] Balance relies predominantly on the activation of specialized reflex actions, which vary from small shifting responses of the ankle or hip to stepping strategies and associated upper-extremity movement to regain center of gravity.[25]

As I discussed in Chapter 2, balance reflexes can be divided into two major classifications, *body-righting reflexes* or *tilting-response reflexes*.[11] These are different reflex actions and will have different training adaptations and benefits. It is important that the appropriate type of reflex is being trained often enough to improve the desired reflex actions. Some sports, such as equestrian events or motorcycle racing, require a combination of both. However, most activities are dominated by the need of one reflex over the other.

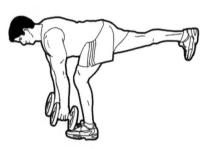

Body-righting reflex training.

Body-righting reflexes, as the one shown in the top figure on this page, tend to dominate when standing or moving on a stable surface, such as when performing a dumbbell, one-leg hip extension, or even as a gymnast performing her routine on a balance beam.[11]

Tilting-response reflexes, as the one shown in the bottom figure, are dominant when the supportive surface can also move beneath us, such as when performing a set of squats on a wobble board or standing on stability disks.[11]

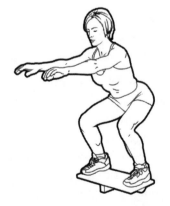

Tilting-response reflex training.

The Stabilization Process

Without stabilization, other elements of technique—particularly the positioning, alignment, and motion—would all be compromised. Stabilization requires the integrated function of all three systems involved in human movement. The passive-skeletal system relies on the active muscular system for holding joint position. The active system, in turn, is reliant on its interdependent relationship with the control-sensorimotor system for reflex actions and commands to control and coordinate the proper activations of the concert of muscle activations needed to provide stability.

The control system provides for *kinesthesia*, which is the conscious awareness of joint position sense and joint movement.[25] Kinesthesia is imperative for stabilization and balance, and results from processing input information to the central nervous system from visual, vestibular, and proprioceptive sources. Proprioception is the cumulative neural input from all the numerous afferent mechanoreceptors in the muscles, joints, connective tissues, and even in the skin.[19] This information then is processed at the appropriate level, and commands are sent to the active system to make the needed adjustments to stabilize the passive system.

In time, *motor programs* of combined movements and stabilization strategies can be performed with little or no conscious thought, and concurrently will require a different level of control. Chek often quotes *Dorland's Medical Dictionary* for the "law of facilitation" that states, "When an impulse has passed once through a certain set of neurons to the exclusion of others, it will tend to take the same course on future occasions, and each time it traverses this path the resistance will become smaller" (p. 47).[11]

This programmable feature of the neuromuscular system should be a part of exercise technique to purposely challenge and improve stability and balance. Improved neuromuscular efficiency is needed for improved stabilization and balance, which are critical components for increases in strength, speed, power, and agility. *Neuromuscular efficiency* can be described as the neuromuscular system's ability to learn, store, and recall motor programs that contain the required force production and reductions, combined with the appropriate stability strategies and balance reflexes. Lack of joint stabilization alters length-tension and force-couple relationships, inhibits recruitment of primary movers, and alters joint mechanics, resulting in faulty movement patterns and compensation.[19]

Stabilization and the Core

Fast or powerful movements cannot take place unless you accomplish adequate stabilization first. Stabilization begins with the spine and is first initiated by the local spinal stabilization subsystem known as the inner unit, or core. Research shows that in healthy individuals, activation of the core muscles occurs before any movement of the body or a body segment.[12, 14, 36] This means core muscles are essential for optimal stabilization and are stimulated any time stability and balance are challenged.

However, this does not mean that simply performing exercises in unstable positions or while standing on unstable apparatus (such as balance boards or stability disks) is enough to develop optimal core function. As discussed in Chapter 1 and in greater detail later in this chapter in the "Breathing" section, that combined respiratory action will help to active and integrate the use of these core muscles for increased stability. There are specific exercises designed to begin core development and integration into movement presented in the first section of Chapter 5, "Strength and Stability Exercises."

Tempo

Probably the most overlooked element of exercise technique is *tempo*, which is defined as the specific movement speed of the body or segments during any given exercise.[1, 2, 27] Tempo for resistance training deals with the actual speed of each repetition. It has traditionally been taught in a nonspecific, very general manner, or given no consideration at all. Occasionally when tempo is mentioned, it is as part of a philosophy that will promote only one tempo that is supposedly best for use on all exercises, for every person, regardless of goal. Basic facts concerning the physiology of contractile units within muscles and general knowledge of neurological function prove these theories to be incorrect.

The Science of Tempo

Mechanoreceptors within the joints, connective tissue, and the muscles themselves monitor not only the muscle force and joint range of motion, but also the speed of force production and the speed of joint motion. This fact alone obviously makes tempo an important element of exercise technique and demonstrates that no one speed can offer the best results for all training goals. Famous Olympic and professional strength coach Charles Poliquin states that "even subtle changes in exercise speed can have profound results for athletes who are looking for above-average gains and performance" (p. 23).[27]

There are better tempos associated with every type of strength gain desired. There are also biomechanical considerations associated with tempo for every exercise for each person's anatomical makeup and individual abilities. Clearly stated, there will be an optimal movement speed on every exercise for each person, depending on the length of their segments, the mobility and stability of the joints involved, and the person's training goals.

Once again we see the overall training goals as a prerequisite for determining appropriate tempo, as they do for all other elements of technique. Tempo also has a significant effect on all other elements, as it can alter the motion, redirect alignment, and cause positioning changes when the body cannot stabilize the duration or speed of movement. Breathing is also closely tied to the tempo and will tend to speed up or slow down with the tempo of the exercise.[1, 2, 4]

Tempo also affects training volume or total time of muscle tension, so it is an important variable for program design considerations. Therefore, when assigning tempos, we must not only think about its possible affects associated with technique, but also its ramifications on determining which energy system and which muscle fiber types will ultimately be targeted. The selected tempo should be consistent with the intensity, sets, reps, and recovery parameters of the particular training phase of the cycle. I will further discuss the specifics of dealing with tempo as a program variable in Chapter 7, "Progressive Program Design."

Tempo Assignment

Placing numbers to the tempo is necessary for estimating the speed of movement. Numerical representations are nothing new; Arthur Jones long ago advised a tempo speed of 4–2 with use of his Nautilus line of equipment. This meant he felt it best to lower the weight to a four count followed by a faster lift of the weight to a two count. This provided more work for the eccentric part of the lift than the concentric, which has debatable benefits, depending on one's goal.

Poliquin, who has probably placed more importance on tempo than any other expert to my knowledge, uses a system developed by Australia's leading strength coach, Ian King.[27] He uses a three-digit number to express tempo. The first number expresses the eccentric phase, the second the isometric phase, and the third number represents the concentric phase of the repetition. The addition of the isometric phase to Jones's two-digit number system is logical, because there must always be a point of nonmovement any time movement is changed by 180 degrees. This led me to develop a four-number system for tempo.[1, 2] There is no real change to King's and Poliquin's system, only the acknowledgement that there is another isometric phase following the concentric phase and before beginning another repetition with the subsequent eccentric phase.

To demonstrate this method, a 4–2–3–1 tempo on a squat would mean to lower the body and bar with a four-second eccentric movement, hold at the bottom for two seconds during the eccentric-isometric phase, press the body and weight load back up with a three-second concentric movement, and then pause for one second at the concentric-isometric phase; then repeat. This would be a nine-second tempo for the squat, which is a very slow repetition speed ideal for certain training goals but inappropriate for others. I often coach to squeeze the muscle during the concentric-isometric phase to maintain muscle tension on certain movements, such as a bicep flexion.

If .5 is used, this denotes a half-second, and a 0 means moving as fast as possible through this phase of the repetition. An example would be a barbell push-press performed at a 10.51. This would mean bringing the weight down quickly with a one-second eccentric movement, exploding through the eccentric-isometric phase, and taking only half a second to press the weight back up during the concentric phase. A second pause is set before beginning the next repetition to reset positioning and regain balance if needed. This type of tempo assignment is used to exploit the stretch reflex of the muscle tendon units and prepare them for more powerful movements. It is good for developing speed-strength and explosive-strength and is designed for use with reduced weight loads as compared to maximal-strength training.

Slower tempos with longer pauses at the eccentric-isometric phase are ideal for developing static- and starting-strength, ans well as maximal-strength gains. The muscle must learn to produce more force and recruit more motor units in absence of the stretch-reflex and plyometric effect.[27] All the resistance training exercises presented in this book give nonspecific tempos with pauses at the eccentric-isometric phase, as I can never be sure who is utilizing this book or what their training needs and goals are. This general tempo assignment will maximize safety, develop static-strength and stabilization, and help to increase the readers' maximal-strength levels. However, this is not always the best tempo for certain specific goals or for different training phases; thus, it should be adjusted accordingly.

Faster tempos are ideal for some of the speed, agility, and power exercises in Chapter 6, as these movements should have been progressed to involve little or no additional loads and are designed to increase the power-producing capability of the muscles by exploiting the stretch-reflex. This also prepares the joints for the similar stresses that will be experienced in a sport or any ballistic life movement. Chapter 7 provides the best examples of use of tempos as they are intentionally altered depending on the exercise and the corresponding training phase.

Take care when increasing tempos, as any increase in tempo must be considered an increase in intensity or load. Just as one would not make a dramatic increase in the amount of weight used on any lift in a week's time, neither should one make dramatic changes in tempo without proper progression.

Breathing

Breathing is another element of technique that has been often oversimplified or completely overlooked. Most every book and instructor recommend breathing, of course, but rarely is there any technically sound method or any scientific rationale associated with the advice.

Breathing is a vital mechanical function requiring the integrated and coordinated action of several muscle groups, regardless of our consciousness of such. In Chapter 1, in the section "The Inner Unit (The Core)," I detail the sequencing of muscle activation required for optimal breathing. If you missed this section or are not clear on this information, you might want to turn back for a quick review before continuing, as the following recommended breathing methods are based on this information about the body's respiratory process.

The Science of Exercise Breathing

The inner unit (or core) has a primary function of respiration, yet it also serves an important secondary role of stabilization. These seemingly different responsibilities of the core are actually logical harmonious functions of its design. With proper breathing technique, the mechanics and associated muscle actions of respiration actually help to stabilize the spine at the same time.[14, 26, 36] It is on the core's intricate design and its unique ability to perform dual functions that these optimal breathing methods are based upon, and this is what makes them another critical element for resistance training technique.

As inhalation begins, the uninhibited contraction of the diaphragm creates a downward pressure on the viscera in the abdominal cavity while simultaneously helping the lungs to draw in more air, expanding the thoracic cavity. The downward pressure forces the contents of the abdominal cavity down, back, and out. The resulting distortion of the viscera combined with the associated neurological reactions of the other core muscles creates joint stiffness of the spine, increased stabilization of the pelvis and sacroiliac joints, and causes a slight distension of the abdominal wall. With the appropriate core muscles activated and pressure within both cavities of the trunk, stabilization is highly internally supported at this point.[10] The figures in Chapter 1, in the section "The Inner Unit (The Core)," illustrate these actions.

Upon full inspiration, an isometric contraction of the transverse abdominus while holding the breath creates what is called the *Valsalva Maneuver*, which provides maximal internal assistance for stabilization of the spine.[40] A person usually experiences this naturally at some level whenever a sudden force is applied to the body that disturbs the center of gravity and challenges posture. We automatically will gasp in a quick breath and hold the breath while reflex responses activate the core and trunk muscles to provide immediate joint stiffness for the spine.

As use of the Valsalva Maneuver is an extremely effective stabilization strategy; it is also short lived as we obviously cannot hold the breath for long durations of time, and even short durations may have risk for certain people. The greatest challenge of maintaining spinal stabilization during respiration and a resisted exercise comes during the exhalation phase. As air is released, both the thoracic and abdominal cavities begin to lose pressure and certain core muscles begin to lose tension, resulting in decreased stability of the spine and pelvis.

The answer to this paradox is through the timely voluntary (or autonomous) contraction of the transverse abdominus. This contraction creates a drawing in of the abdominal wall and tightening of the thoracolumbar fasciae. This helps to maintain pressure within the abdominal cavity and presses the contents of the viscera back, down, and up. The backward pressure of the viscera signals or maintains the reflex activation of the multifidi and associated deep erector muscles of the spine, creating joint stiffness.[14, 36, 40] The downward pressure has a similar effect on the muscles of the pelvic floor, stabilizing the pelvis and sacroiliac joints from the inside out.

The upward pressure helps to maintain pressure in the thoracic cavity that is being lost during exhalation. The drawing in of the abdominal wall is somewhat proportional to the level of exhalation. It should not, however, result in a concave distortion of the abdomen, nor should a complete exhalation be performed for exercises in need of higher levels of stabilization. Another benefit for maintaining intraabdominal pressure is the hydraulic-lift mechanism that relieves compressive forces placed on the vertebral disks in the presence of flexon forces.

Breathing for Resistance Training

To put this breathing method into practice, begin with the core activation exercises discussed in the beginning of Chapter 5. With most exercise movements, try inhaling during the eccentric phase, allowing the abdominal wall to slightly distend so as not to inhibit diaphragmatic action or recruitment of scalene musculature. However, be sure not to lose all abdominal tension or allow any associated movement of the spine, and avoid any elevation of the scapula. During the eccentric-isometric phase where stability is typically needed the most, hold the breath and perform the Valsalva Maneuver by activating the transverse abdominus.

As you begin the concentric phase of the movement, start to exhale while drawing in the abdominal wall by further contracting the transverse abdominus. During the concentric-isometric phase, stop exhaling your air short of fully emptying the lungs in order to keep some pressure in the thoracic cavity and maintain posture. A tight contraction of the transverse abdominus, short of concaving the abdominal wall and an isometric contraction of the outer abdominal muscles can be felt at this point. Then inhale, release tension of the transverse abdominus so as not to inhibit diaphragm contraction, and begin the eccentric movement of the next repetition.

For certain exercises, you will reverse the breathing because of inverse needs of maximal stability demands for the particular movement. These breathing methods will take time to master and integrate into every exercise. Try beginning with slower tempos for your exercises to best train proper core activation for each movement. In time and with consistent use, this method will become a natural action of neuromuscular control and will dramatically increase the overall effectiveness and safety of your training. Proper activation of the core muscles also eliminates the need for weight belts. This possibly obsolete support gear has been questioned for its ability to adequately add stability and is even seen as detrimental to developing core strength by several experts.[14, 15, 33]

Breathing Relationships

Breathing has an obvious relationship to stability but can also affect other elements of technique. Because breathing affects posture, positioning is closely linked to the ability to perform proper and consistent breathing mechanics. Inefficient breathing patterns will quickly increase the heart rate and reduce oxygen supply to the muscles and brain, increasing risks and reducing overall performance. If stability and positioning are compromised as a result of faulty breathing methods, alignment also might be compromised; the motion will then be altered, and accomplishing the training goal will not be possible at the optimal level. Breathing coincides with tempo; thus, you must adjust it depending on the tempo demands of the exercise and the phase of the training cycle. In short, incorporation and practice of efficient breathing methods is a critical element of exercise technique.

Summary

Exercise technique, particularly with resistance training, is critical for ensuring safety and maximizing efficiency. Technique should be based on the designed structure and functions of the human body. This means incorporating the study of the sciences involved in human movement such as anatomy, kinesiology, and physiology. Other scientific considerations, such as biomechanics and physics, should also be a part of developing sound training techniques. After reviewing all this data and the practical experiences of numerous experts, certain elements of technique common to any resistance training exercise have emerged. I have categorized these elements of technique as the overall goals, exercise motion, alignment, positioning, stabilization, tempo, and breathing.

Identifying general goals, specific goals, individual needs, and considerations for the neurological and musculoskeletal systems are all important for overall goal determination. The overall training goals will automatically dictate certain options for all other elements of exercise technique. The overall goals will also influence several variables of program design as well, such as the load, volume, recovery, and frequency an exercise is performed. Therefore, it is important to clearly identify all training goals before selecting any exercise or applying any technique.

After the training goals are clearly understood, the next element in exercise technique to consider is the motion of the exercise. The first prerequisite is choosing the appropriate type of motion that provides the correct path of motion to accomplish your training goals. Next comes setting the desired ROM through analysis of the musculoskeletal system, the effects of internal and external forces, and the control abilities of the sensorimotor system. Finally, evaluate the specificity of the motion to see if the movement itself is of some value toward further progression of our training goals. If the movement accomplishes a desired goal or serves a present need, it is considered functional for this goal.

Alignment can be defined as matching the pull of the muscles in opposition to the pull or push of the resistance. Alignment is interdependent with the goal, the exercise motion, and positioning. It also affects all other elements of technique. Alignment must start with considering the overall training goals; it must be accomplished through positioning and be appropriate for the type, path, and range of exercise motion. Alignment choices affect the stabilization and balance demands and can inadvertently be altered when tempos or breathing methods are changed. Maintaining proper alignment throughout an exercise is a critical element of technique.

Positioning is the precise manner in which you set the body and place all of its segments before and during any resisted exercise. Positioning is a vital element of technique that is interdependent with all training goals, relies on the specifics of alignment, must be appropriate for the motion, and must be able to be stabilized for it to be maximally efficient and safe. Although the positioning of all parts of the body is important in any resistance exercise, particular attention should be given to the spine and pelvis. Optimal posture is usually the best position to work in, as this positioning allows for the best length-tension relationships of all associated pelvic and trunk muscles and inevitably affects the function of the entire kinetic chain. Only when the exercise is designed to target the outer-trunk musculature or purposely involve spinal movements is optimal posture manipulated.

Stabilization is the internal ability to control all desired movement or nonmovement of the body and its segments, in response to the environment or changes in center of gravity. Stabilization can be a static, dynamic, or balance demand. Resistance training programs should include techniques that implement all these stabilization demands, as most life and sports movements will also require them. Balance is the ability to maintain one's center of gravity over his or her base of support. Balance can be divided into two basic reflex actions: body-righting reflexes and tilting-response reflexes. Either can be trained by selecting the appropriate exercise and by applying the proper techniques. Stabilization affects all other elements of technique and is a prerequisite for power.

Tempo is defined as the specific movement speed of the body or its segments during any given exercise. Tempo is often overlooked as an independent training stimulus, but has great potential for bringing about different training adaptations. Different tempos are more appropriate for different training goals. A four-digit number can be used to express tempo and specify the desired speed of contraction at each phase of a repetition. Tempo is dependent on overall goals, it affects all other elements of technique, and is particularly linked to breathing mechanics. Because tempo directly affects the muscle's total amount of time under tension, it is also a component of training volume and a variable of program design.

Breathing is another important and often overlooked element of exercise technique. Breathing methods should be based on the design and functions of the respiratory musculature and the structures in which they are anchored. The local spinal stabilization system known as the inner unit, or the core, has the unique ability to perform the dual functions of respiration and stabilization and is the basis for breathing technique. There are optimal breathing methods that coincide with tempo for every exercise, which will increase stabilization and assist with positioning, and can affect the alignment, overall motion, and ultimately the goal. Optimal breathing increases the efficiency and safety of any resistance training exercise movement.

Strength and Stability Exercises

This chapter will present several exercises for the core, trunk, and lower and upper body that are designed to increase levels of strength and stability. The selection of exercises varies in the stability and balance demands to provide a well-balanced collection of challenging movements for each area of the body. Some exercises have high degrees of neural challenge and provide increased amounts of proprioception. Other exercises are less complex and allow for neural availability to recruit a greater amount of motor units and muscle fiber for the targeted muscle to accomplish maximal strength and hypertrophy goals.

We begin with exercises designed to develop core strength and control. It is critical to master these core-activation and breathing techniques because they are integrated into every exercise thereafter. Exercises for the outer trunk muscles are presented next. They will progress from exercises designed for increasing spinal movement through isolated trunk actions to exercises that focus on static stability training, then finally to integrated trunk movements. Then we'll discuss lower and upper body exercises.

These sections provide a good supply of traditional isolated movements, but definitely focus more on compound movements and contain numerous exercises designed for strengthening general movement patterns such as squatting, lunging, pulling, and pushing. Many of these exercises also demand high levels of internal stabilization and balance, which, combined with the core and trunk work, will improve overall strength and stability that assist with development of all bio-motor abilities.

Here are some suggestions for resistance training:

* Always begin with a 5- to 10-minute general warm-up.
* Perform some active stretching for the entire body before—or as part of—the exercise routine.
* Always do a specific warm-up for each exercise by performing an initial low-intensity set for each exercise with the desired path, range, and speed of motion in place.
* Allow for proper motor learning before progressing to higher-intensity loads.
* Be sure to properly integrate the core activation and breathing techniques for each exercise.
* Use the tempos that are appropriate for the overall training goals and consistent with the training phases.
* Train with high effort, good focus, and exceptional technique to achieve maximal results with minimum risk.

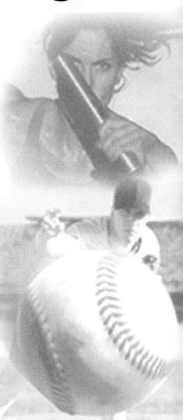

Core Exercises

Four-Point Core Activation

This exercise is designed with the most neurologically advantageous position to learn core activation and develop transversus abdominal (TA) strength. The direct gravitational pull on the viscera provides the best proprioception for activation of the core muscles by encouraging a full lengthening of the TA prior to contraction. Working directly against this gravitational pull forces the TA to exert effort against a maximal amount of internal resistance. This makes it a great strengthening exercise for the TA without integrating any limb movement or activating other muscle groups.

Alignment and Positioning

Assume a hands-and-knees position with the knees placed directly below the hips and hands directly below the shoulders; slightly bend the elbows.

Position the spine in posture, and hold the head in neutral with the eyes looking straight down.

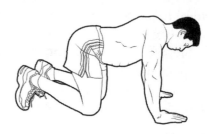

Motion and Stabilization

Draw a deep breath and allow the abdominal area to distend and chest to expand without losing the posture position of the spine.

Slowly breathe out and contract the transversus abdominis by focusing on pulling the belly button up toward the spine as far as possible.

Exhale all remaining air while continuing to pull the abdominal area up and in. Hold, then slowly inhale and repeat.

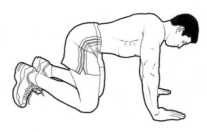

Two-Point Core Activation

This exercise is designed to continue development of core activation and transversus abdominal strength. The two-point position not only requires much more neural demand for balance; you also need additional trunk, shoulder, and hip muscle actions for stabilization. These additional requirements will make it a much more difficult exercise for controlling core activation and achieving full contractions of the transversus abdominis. If this proves too difficult, you can go to a three-point position until ready to progress back to this exercise.

Alignment and Positioning

Start on the hands and knees with one knee placed directly below the hip and the opposite hand directly below the shoulder while holding the contra-lateral leg and arm straight out from the body.

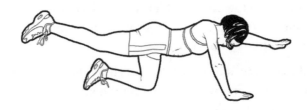

Position the spine in posture, and hold the head in neutral with the eyes looking straight down.

Motion and Stabilization

Draw a deep breath and allow the abdominal area to distend and chest to expand without losing the posture position of the spine.

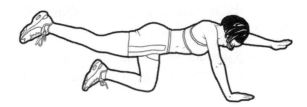

Slowly breathe out and contract the transversus abdominis by focusing on pulling the belly button up toward the spine as far as possible.

Exhale all remaining air while continuing to pull the abdominal area up and in. Hold, then slowly inhale and repeat.

Quadraplex

The quadraplex is simply a two-point core-activation exercise with added movement of the arm and contra-lateral leg. The required muscle actions of the shoulder and hip to move and decelerate the limbs, along with the increased demand on the trunk and core muscles for stabilization, make this exercise an advanced progression in core training. Keep in mind that you must focus as much on what body parts should not be moving as on controlling those in voluntary motion.

Alignment and Positioning

Start on the hands and knees with one knee placed directly below the hip and the opposite hand directly below the shoulder, while placing the contra-lateral leg and arm straight out from the body and just off the ground.

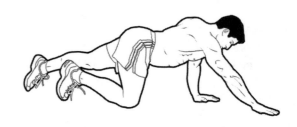

Slowly draw a deep breath and allow the abdominal area to distend while maintaining neutral posture in the spine and the head.

Motion and Stabilization

Slowly exhale and draw the belly button toward the spine; raise the arm and opposite leg without losing the posture position of the spine.

Hold the top position while continuing to contract the transversus abdominis and stabilizing the spine posture.

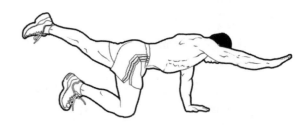

Slowly inhale and lower the leg and arm while allowing the abdominals to slightly distend and chest to expand. Always maintain posture throughout the exercise; repeat.

Standing Core Activation

This exercise trains core activation in a vertical position. Standing positions are slightly more challenging than the seated versions of this exercise because the center of gravity has been raised. You should learn this exercise before any rowing, pushing, pulling, trunk stabilization, and arm exercises are performed in standing positions. A similar level of core activation is a required part of technique for any of those exercises, so it should be mastered before progressing to more complex exercises. This exercise does not have to be performed in a gym; it can be practiced any time you find yourself in a standing or seated position.

Alignment and Positioning

Stand in the posture position with the feet set hip-width apart and pointed straight ahead.

Slightly flex the hip and knee and draw a deep breath, allowing the abdominal area to slightly distend and the chest to expand, with the spine held firm in posture; avoid any shrugging of the shoulder blades.

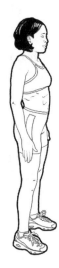

Motion and Stabilization

Slowly exhale and draw the belly button toward the spine while maintaining optimal posture.

Hold this position while continuing to exhale, contracting the transversus abdominis, and stabilizing the spine.

Slowly inhale while allowing the abdominals to slightly distend and chest to expand, keeping the scapula depressed; perform the desired repetitions.

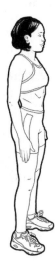

One-Point Core Activation

This exercise trains core activation in a vertical position with only one anchor point. Reducing your anchor will make this exercise more challenging than the two-point standing versions making it more difficult for core activation. This position also requires more stabilization of the ankle and hip of the stationary leg. You should learn this exercise before any rowing, pushing, pulling, trunk stabilization, and arm exercises are performed in standing one-point positions. You should also master this before adding lunges, because they will require similar core activation and overall stabilization while on one leg.

Alignment and Positioning

Stand in the posture position with one foot set midline of the body and the toes pointed straight ahead.

Slightly bend the hip and knee; then draw a deep breath, allowing the abdominal area to slightly distend and chest to expand with the spine held firm in posture and avoiding any shrugging of the shoulder blades.

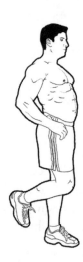

Motion and Stabilization

Slowly exhale and draw the belly button toward the spine while maintaining optimal posture.

Hold this position while continuing to exhale and contracting the transversus abdominis, as well as stabilizing the spine.

Slowly inhale while allowing the abdominals to slightly distend and chest to expand, keeping the scapula depressed. Perform the desired repetitions.

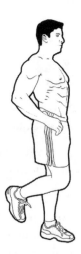

Supine Core Activation

This exercise trains core activation in the supine position. This is the most difficult body angle to get proprioception for activating and strengthening the transversus abdominis because the gravitational pull on the viscera assists with its action. However, the supine position is ideal for challenging the action of the diaphragm muscle. Contraction of the diaphragm results in a downward pull on the entire contents of the abdominal cavity, which produces a degree of abdominal distension that will be directly resisted by gravity. Learn and teach this exercise before any pressing, pulling, leg raising, or trunk exercises are performed in supine positions, because a similar core activation is a part of technique for those exercises.

Alignment and Positioning

Lay supine while in good posture, a natural arch in the lower spine, the knees bent, and feet set comfortably on the floor.

Draw a deep breath, forcing the abdominal area to slightly distend upward and the chest to expand with the spine held in posture and avoiding any shrugging of the shoulder blades.

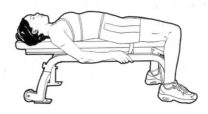

Motion and Stabilization

Slowly exhale and draw the belly button toward the spine while maintaining the natural arch in the lower spine.

Hold this position while continuing to exhale and contracting the transversus abdominis, and stabilizing the spine.

Slowly inhale while allowing the abdominals to slightly distend and the chest to expand, keeping the scapula depressed; perform the desired repetitions.

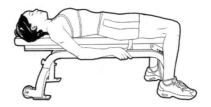

Supine Core Activation with Bent Leg Raises

This exercise continues to train core activation in the supine position. The added action of the hip flexor muscles combined with the inertia of the moving leg makes this exercise substantially more demanding on the core and trunk muscles for stabilization of the spine while continuing to perform proper respiratory functions. As with any supine exercise, the upward distension of the viscera is directly resisted by gravity, making it great for strengthening diaphragmatic action. Learn and teach this exercise before any pressing, pulling, leg raising, or trunk exercises are performed in supine positions, as core activation is necessary for those exercises.

Alignment and Positioning

Lay supine while in good posture, a natural arch in the lower spine, the knees bent 90 degrees, and feet in a neutral position.

Draw a deep breath while lowering the leg and allowing the abdominals to slightly distend upward, keeping the scapula depressed and the spine neutral.

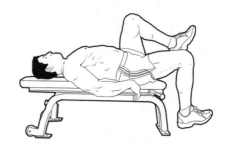

Motion and Stabilization

Slowly exhale and draw the belly button toward the spine while raising the leg back up and maintaining the natural arch in the lower spine.

Hold this position while continuing to exhale, contracting the transversus abdominis, and stabilizing the spine. Then repeat.

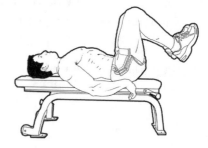

Trunk Exercises

Incline Bench, Trunk Flexion

This exercise targets the abdominal and oblique musculature and trains flexion of the spine in a gravity-assisted position. The incline angle and stable bench allow the lifter to achieve maximal spinal flexion more easily. You can vary the amount of incline to increase or decrease resistance as desired. Altering leg positions to increase or decrease hip flexor involvement is also a viable option, depending on the lifter's ability and goals.

Alignment and Positioning

Lay supine on the inclined bench with the feet braced lightly on the anchor pad or wall, with the hips and knees bent about 60 and 90 degrees, respectively.

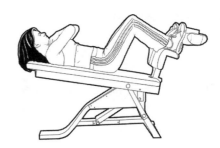

Spread the legs so the feet are angled out about 45 degrees or are at about 2 and 10 o'clock.

Place the fists under the chin and begin with a full breath of air, the shoulders just off the bench, and tension in the abdominals.

Motion and Stabilization

Slowly exhale and pull the ribs toward the pelvis, attempting to move one vertebra at a time.

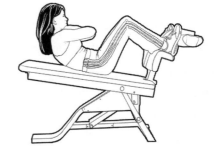

Hold the top position while continuing to exhale, contracting the abdominals, and relaxing the neck.

Slowly inhale while lowering the torso to the starting position, maintaining the head position and tension in the abdominals.

Swiss Ball, Trunk Flexion

The Swiss ball is excellent for trunk training. The ball's shape and yielding surface allow for much greater range of motion when beginning in a position of spinal extension. This exercise targets the abdominal and oblique musculature and trains flexion of the spine while requiring greater core and trunk muscle demand for moderate balance challenges. You can apply different angles of resistance by simply repositioning the body on the ball. Shifting the body down on the ball creates more of an incline angle, decreasing resistance. Shifting more of the lower back and pelvis on the ball flattens out the angle of pull and adds more resistance because of a longer resistance arm.

Alignment and Positioning

Lay supine on the ball with the feet spread and placed on the floor.

Adjust desired angle on the ball and let the spine bend back over the ball as available and comfortable to the spine.

Place the fists just under the chin and begin with a full breath of air and tension in the abdominals.

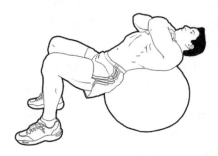

Motion and Stabilization

Slowly exhale and pull the ribs toward the pelvis, attempting to move one vertebra at a time.

Hold the top position while continuing to exhale, contracting the abdominals, and relaxing the neck.

Slowly inhale while lowering the torso to the starting position and maintaining the head position and tension in the abdominals.

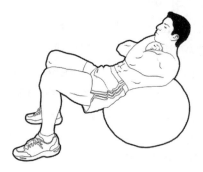

Flat Bench, Reverse Trunk Flexion

This exercise targets the abdominal and oblique musculature and trains flexion of the spine in a reverse movement. The reverse trunk flexion contracts the abdominal muscle from an opposite insertion-to-origin pattern, as compared to trunk flexion exercises. This movement also develops an initial activation of the lower fibers of the *rectus abdominis* and creates a greater degree of flexion in the lumbar region, and less in the thoracic region, than trunk flexion. You can use different angles of incline or decline with an adjustable bench to increase or decrease resistance.

Alignment and Positioning

Lay supine on the bench with the hips and knees bent at about 90 degrees.

Anchor the body with the arms, and begin with the head just off the pad to target the neck and trunk flexors.

Posteriorly tilt the pelvis to flatten the lower back; begin with a full breath of air and tension on the abdominals.

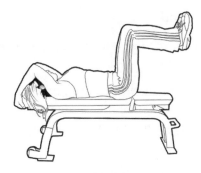

Motion and Stabilization

Slowly exhale and pull the pelvis toward the ribs, attempting to move one vertebra at a time.

Hold the top position while continuing to exhale, contracting the abdominals, and holding the head in position.

Slowly inhale while lowering the pelvis to the starting position and maintaining tension in the abdominals—your head can rest on the bench at any time if needed.

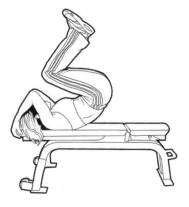

Swiss Ball, Reverse Trunk Flexion

This exercise targets the abdominal and oblique musculature and trains flexion of the spine in a reverse movement. Contracting the abdominal muscle from an insertion to origin pattern might develop an initial and possibly increased activation of the lower fibers of the rectus abdominis. Use of the ball also requires different core and trunk muscle recruitment to correct balance challenges. You can apply different angles of resistance by simply repositioning the body on the ball. Shifting the body down on the ball creates more of an incline angle increasing resistance; shifting more of the lower back and pelvis on the ball decreases the resistance.

Alignment and Positioning

Lay supine on the ball with the hips and knees bent at about 90 degrees.

Anchor the body with the arms and begin with the spine pressed against and extended over the ball (as available and comfortable to the spine).

Begin with a full breath of air, head held in neutral, and tension in the abdominals.

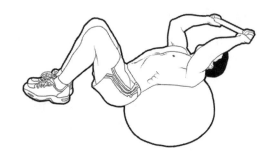

Motion and Stabilization

Slowly exhale and pull the pelvis toward the ribs, moving one vertebra at a time.

Hold the top position while continuing to exhale, contracting the abdominals, and holding the head in position.

Slowly inhale while lowering the pelvis to the starting position and maintaining tension in the abdominals.

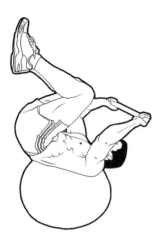

Incline Bench, Trunk Extension

This exercise targets the spinal extensors particularly of the thoracic region with some lumber and hip extensors assistance. Using a stable bench allows the lifter to more specifically control how much and where spinal movement occurs. Keep in mind it often is very difficult for some individuals to produce extension of the mid and upper back without hyperextending the lower back. Variations in the amount of incline can be made as desired to increase or decrease resistance. Altering leg positions to increase or decrease hip extensor involvement is also a viable option.

Alignment and Positioning

Lay prone on the inclined bench with the legs spread comfortably and feet braced against the floor.

Place the arms against the body, out to the side, or overhead depending on desired resistance and abilities.

Begin with a full breath of air and the chest just off the bench with tension on the extensors.

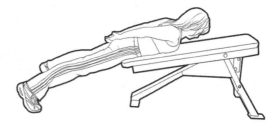

Motion and Stabilization

Slowly exhale, activate the core, and pull the shoulder blades together and down while moving one thoracic vertebra at a time.

Extend up and back as far as possible without hyperextending the lower back and hold the top position.

Slowly inhale while lowering the torso to the starting position and maintaining the head position and tension in the extensors; then repeat.

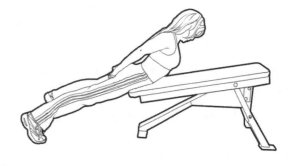

Swiss Ball, Trunk Extension

This exercise targets the spinal extensors, particularly those in the thoracic region with some hip extensors assistance. Using a ball can increase the range of motion if beginning in a position of spinal flexion. The ball also requires some different core, trunk, and hip musculature recruitment to correct for righting and tilting response reflexes and balance challenges. You can make variations in the angle and desired weight load by adjusting body position on the ball. Altering leg positions to increase or decrease hip extensor involvement is also a viable option, depending on the lifter's ability and goals.

Alignment and Positioning

Lay prone on the ball with the legs spread comfortably and feet braced against the floor.

Bend the spine comfortably over the ball and place the arms against the body, out to the side, or overhead, depending on desired resistance.

Begin with a full breath of air and the chest just off the ball with tension on the extensors.

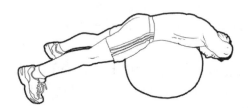

Motion and Stabilization

Slowly exhale, activate the core, and pull the shoulder blades together and back, moving one thoracic vertebra at a time.

Extend up and back as far as possible without hyperextending the lower back; hold the top position.

Slowly inhale while lowering the torso to the starting position while maintaining the head position and tension in the extensors; then repeat.

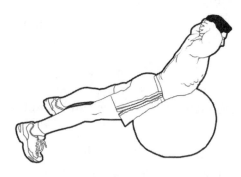

Swiss Ball, Trunk Lateral Flexion

This exercise iso-laterally targets the quadratus lumborum, internal obliques, and portions of the external obliques, rectus abdominis, and spinal extensors to the side of movement. Using the ball can increase the range of motion if beginning in a position of lateral flexion to the opposite side. It also requires some different core, trunk, and hip musculature recruitment to correct for righting and tilting response reflexes and balance challenges. You can make variations in the angle and desired weight load by adjusting body position on the ball. Altering leg position to increase or decrease hip abductor involvement is also a viable option, depending on the lifter's ability and goals.

Alignment and Positioning

Lay on your side over the ball with the top leg placed in front of the body, and the bottom leg straight and slightly behind the body.

Bend the spine comfortably over the ball; place the bottom arm on the side; and place the top arm against the body or overhead, depending on the desired resistance. Begin with a full breath of air.

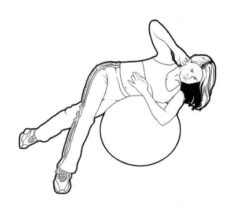

Motion and Stabilization

Slowly exhale; activate the core and pull the lower ribs toward the crest of the pelvic girdle, attempting to move laterally, one vertebra at a time.

Pull the trunk up and over as far as possible without flexing or extending the spine, continuing to exhale.

Hold; then slowly inhale while lowering the torso to the starting position, while maintaining the head position and tension in the lateral flexors.

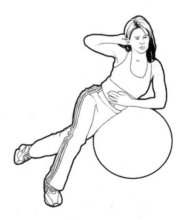

Seated Trunk Rotation

This exercise is designed to introduce rotational movements to the spine. It allows the lifter to begin training isolated spinal rotation with proper posture and integrated core activation. The rotational movement is not directly resisted, making this a good active stretching exercise. The seated position stabilizes the pelvis, allowing you to assess present active ranges of available motion. You should note that while in optimal posture, normal trunk rotation is listed at only 30 degrees. Attempting to increase range farther through use of forces or speed of movement can be detrimental to the disks and connective tissues of the spine.

Alignment and Positioning

Sit in good posture with the back unsupported and the pelvis set to provide a natural arch in the lower back.

Place the hands behind the ears, elbows pointed straight out; then pull the shoulder blades together.

Draw a deep breath, allowing the abdominal area to slightly distend and chest to expand, with the spine held in posture; avoid any shrugging of the shoulder blades.

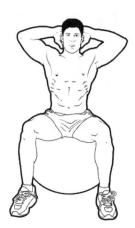

Motion and Stabilization

Slowly exhale; activate the core and rotate the torso while avoiding flexing or extending of the spine.

Twist as far as possible; hold this position while continuing to exhale and activating the core muscles.

Slowly inhale while rotating to the starting position, allowing the abdominals to slightly distend and keeping the scapula depressed.

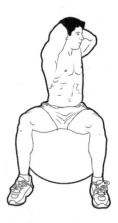

Supine Trunk Rotation

This exercise is designed to begin loaded, isolated rotation of the spine. It allows the lifter to strengthen the external obliques and associated trunk rotators in a stabilized position. It is important to develop the strength and control of these muscles before progressing to more integrated movements. Once integrated movements are required, the body will compensate with other joints and muscles for any weakness or lack of movement in spinal rotation.

Alignment and Positioning

Lay supine on the floor with the feet braced lightly on a low bench or chair.

Place one leg over the other and rotate the pelvis and legs about 35 degrees with the sternum still facing up.

Place the bottom hand on the side and the other hand behind the head, and begin with the shoulders slightly off the ground and a full breath of air.

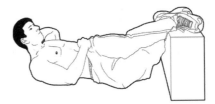

Motion and Stabilization

Slowly exhale; activate the core and pull the rib cage slightly up and over to align with the pelvis, keeping the head in a neutral position.

Hold the top position while continuing to exhale and contracting the core, abdominal, and oblique muscles.

Slowly inhale while lowering the torso to the starting position, while maintaining the head position and tension in the abdominals and obliques.

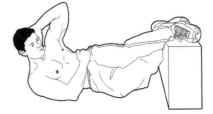

Cable Trunk Rotation with Pulls

This exercise is designed to teach integrated and loaded rotation of the spine. It targets and strengthens the external obliques and associated trunk rotators in a standing position, while integrating lower body musculature for stabilization and posterior upper body muscles for the pulling movement. This exercise directly targets the posterior oblique subsystem. This integrated subsystem of posterior trunk and lower body musculature forms an active sling that assists with pelvic and spinal stabilization, propels the body during gait, and decelerates the trunk and limbs during powerful rotational movements. Teaching the body how to produce and reduce rotational forces in this manner will be critical before progressing to faster, more ballistic exercises involving spinal rotation.

Alignment and Positioning

Stand in a lunge position, with the back leg straight, lean the trunk forward placing the weight over the lead leg while maintaining good posture.

Grasp the handle with the hand opposite of the lead leg and begin with the arm straight and perpendicular to the trunk, with the elbow out.

Draw a deep breath and begin with the trunk rotated, keeping the pelvis and head aligned straight.

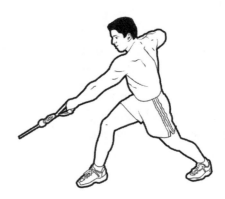

Motion and Stabilization

Slowly exhale; activate the core and rotate the spine while pulling the arm out and back and keeping the head and pelvis straight.

Rotate the spine and pull the arm back, while continuing to exhale and contracting the core muscles.

Hold; then slowly inhale while rotating the torso back around and down to the starting position and maintaining the head and pelvic positions.

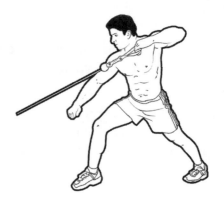

Cable Trunk Rotation with Press

This exercise is also designed to begin teaching integrated and loaded rotation of the spine. It targets and strengthens the external obliques and associated trunk rotators in a standing position, while integrating lower body musculature for stabilization, and anterior upper body muscles for pulling movement. This exercise directly targets the actions of the anterior oblique subsystem. This integrated subsystem of anterior trunk and lower body musculature is used for powerful rotational movements such as throwing or swinging implements. It is also highly active in the swing phase of gait. Teaching the body how to produce rotational forces in this manner is critical before progressing to faster, more ballistic exercises involving spinal rotation.

Alignment and Positioning

Grasp the upper pulley handle and step forward with the opposite leg into a lunge position, the back leg straight, the trunk leaned forward, and in good posture.

Position the arm up, aligned perpendicular to the trunk with the elbow out.

Begin with the spine rotated with the feet, pelvis, and head aligned straight; draw a deep breath.

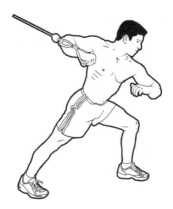

Motion and Stabilization

Slowly exhale while rotating the trunk, pressing the handle down and around, and keeping the elbow pointed out with the head and pelvis straight.

Continue to rotate the spine and press the hand down while continuing to exhale and contract the core muscles.

Hold; then slowly inhale while rotating the torso back around and up to the starting position, maintaining head and pelvic position.

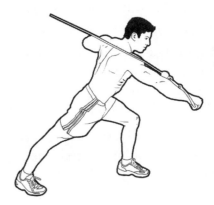

Lower Body Exercises

Flat Bench, Bent-Leg Hip Flexion

This exercise is designed to strengthen the hip flexor musculature and can also challenge the abdominals and neck flexors. However, performing this movement on a flat bench requires only minor levels of stabilization strength of the abdominals; allowing the head to rest whenever needed will ensure the exercise is not terminated because of neck flexor weakness. Moving only one leg at a time and bending the knee to reduce the lever arm of the resistance also allow for a lighter beginning weight load on the hip flexors, as compared to straight-leg versions. Progress to straight-leg, double-leg, incline bench, or Swiss ball versions when you desire more of a challenge.

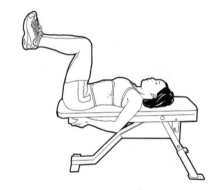

Alignment and Positioning

Lay supine on a flat bench in good posture with the hands resting on the bench or across the trunk.

Pull both legs up and bend them approximately 90 degrees.

Begin with the head slightly off the bench, with the chin slightly tucked.

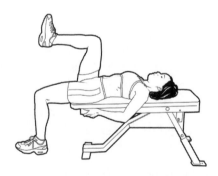

Motion and Stabilization

Slowly inhale while lowering one leg until the thigh is parallel with the body, or as low as possible while maintaining posture and head position.

Hold at the bottom position; then slowly exhale, activate the core, and pull the leg up to the starting position while maintaining head and spinal position. Repeat with same or opposite leg.

Note: Let the head rest whenever needed so neck weakness does not inhibit strengthening of the hip flexors.

Incline Bench, Straight-Leg Hip Flexion

This exercise targets strengthening of the hip flexor musculature, as well as challenges the abdominals and neck flexors. By straightening the leg you automatically increase the load and add the passive tension of the hamstrings and gastrocs (when foot is flexed) to the resistance. For people with tight hamstrings, this can be a significant and even prohibitive amount of resistance. You can use slight bends in the knee in such cases to keep an optimal amount of active motion. You can progress to inclined angles, alternate legs, perform piston movements, or choose double-leg and Swiss ball versions when you desire more challenge.

Alignment and Positioning

Lay supine on an inclined bench in good posture with the hands anchoring on the handle or top of the bench.

Pull both legs up, one bent and the other one straight with foot flexed.

Begin with the head slightly off the bench with the chin slightly tucked.

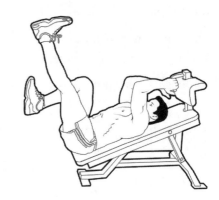

Motion and Stabilization

Slowly inhale while lowering the straight leg until the thigh is parallel with the body, or as low as possible while maintaining posture and head position.

Hold at the bottom position; then slowly exhale, activate the core, and pull the leg up to the starting position while maintaining the head and spinal positions.

Let the head rest whenever needed so neck weakness does not inhibit strengthening of the hip flexors.

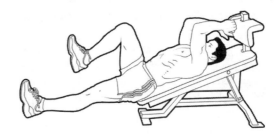

Swiss Ball, Double-Leg Hip Flexion

This exercise further targets strengthening of the hip flexor musculature and increases the challenge of the abdominals and neck flexors. Using a Swiss ball increases demand on the core and trunk muscles, which helps to overcome balancing challenges and meet stabilization requirements. You must learn single-leg versions before attempting the double-leg exercise. You can implement increased angles and greater loads for more resistance by simply adjusting the body down on the ball. Neck flexor strength is a prerequisite for this exercise, as the head cannot be easily rested at any time during the movement.

Alignment and Positioning

Lay supine on a Swiss ball in good posture with the hands anchoring on a stable object.

Pull both legs up with both legs straight and feet flexed.

Begin with the head held in alignment with the spine and chin slightly tucked.

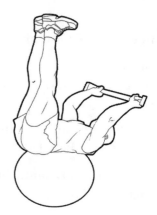

Motion and Stabilization

Slowly inhale; lower the legs until the thighs are parallel with the body, or as low as possible while maintaining posture and head position.

Hold at the bottom position; then slowly exhale, activate the core, and pull the legs up to the starting position while maintaining the head and spinal positions.

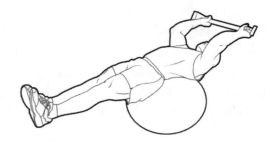

Inclined Bench, Double-Leg Hip Extension

This exercise targets the glutes and hamstring musculature. Besides these hip extensors, the spinal erectors are challenged for stabilization requirements. If available, you can also use special hyper-benches to increase range of motion for this exercise. An external rotation of the hip is presented on this exercise to further activate the gluteus muscle, but is not necessary or always desired for some goals. You can also add resistance while holding a med ball between the feet. This exercise might not be appropriate for some individuals with abdominal discomfort or lower back problems.

Alignment and Positioning

Lay prone on a bench in good posture with the hands anchored under the bench.

Position the hips on the edge of the bench with the legs straight and feet just touching the ground.

Begin with the head held in alignment with the spine and draw a deep breath.

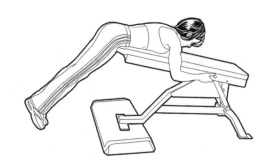

Motion and Stabilization

Slowly exhale; activate the core and lift the legs while twisting the feet out until legs are parallel with the body, or as high as possible while maintaining posture and head position.

Hold at the top position; then slowly inhale and lower the legs to the starting position while maintaining the head and spinal positions.

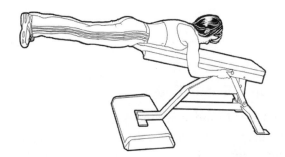

45-Degree Hip Extension

This exercise is designed to target the glutes and hamstring musculature. The spinal erectors are also challenged as stabilizers and will be strengthened along with the hip extensors. Slight external rotation of the hips is presented in this exercise to further activate the gluteus muscle, but is not necessary or always advisable, particularly for those with previous lateral collateral ligament injuries. Because the knee is forced into a locked position against direct load, larger individuals—or someone with hyper-mobile or unstable knees—should not use this device. Also, heavy additional loads are not suggested as knee instability can result over time. Barbell and dumbbell hip extension exercises are better options for these individuals.

Alignment and Positioning

Position the hips in line to the top edge of the pad with the hips and feet slightly rotated out.

Place the hands just behind the ears, and pull the shoulder blades together with the spine and head in good posture.

Exhale all air and activate the core by pulling the belly button toward the spine.

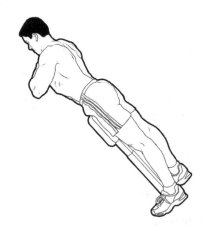

Motion and Stabilization

Slowly inhale and lower the trunk to the maximum of 90 degrees or as low as the hamstrings will allow while maintaining proper posture and head position.

Hold at the bottom position; then slowly exhale, activating the core and pulling the torso back up to the starting position while maintaining the head and spinal positions.

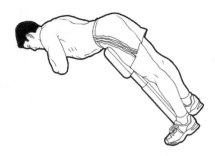

Barbell Hip Extension

This exercise is designed to further strengthen the glutes and hamstring musculature. The spinal erectors are also challenged as stabilizers and will be strengthened along with the hip extensors. Using barbells, dumbbells, or other free-weight loads better conditions the lifter to the functional lifts he might need to perform in certain life activities. This exercise, performed with the proper lifting technique, is a highly valuable movement to practice, particularly for those with lower back problems or weakness.

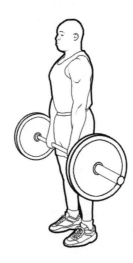

Alignment and Positioning

Position the feet straight ahead and directly under the hips, with knees slightly bent.

Place the hands on the bar at shoulder width at alternate grip and lift the bar into position with the spine in good posture.

Begin with the shoulders back, spine and head in posture; exhale and activate the core.

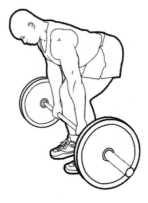

Motion and Stabilization

Slowly inhale and push the hips back while lowering the trunk as low as the hamstrings will allow, maintaining proper posture and keeping the bar close to the body.

Hold at the bottom position; then slowly exhale, activating the core and pulling the torso back up to the starting position while relaxing the arms and maintaining proper posture.

Dumbbell, One-Leg Hip Extension

This exercise is designed to strengthen the glutes and hamstring musculature, challenge the hamstrings' active flexibility, and improve balance. The ankle and hip of the stationary leg have a high demand to provide stabilization. The spinal erectors are also highly challenged as stabilizers to avoid flexion or rotation of the spine. This exercise is an advanced movement ideal for those looking for improved balance, hip and ankle stabilization, active flexibility training, and overall glute and hamstring development. People with either low hamstring flexibility or lack of good balance reflexes might need to improve in these areas before performing this exercise.

Alignment and Positioning

Position the foot of the stationary leg straight ahead and hold the other leg up in a crane position.

Hold the dumbbells relaxed at the side of the body, balance, and assume good posture.

Begin with the shoulders back, spine and head in posture; exhale and activate the core.

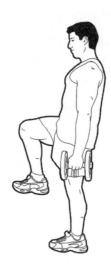

Motion and Stabilization

Slowly inhale; pull the leg down and slowly reach back and straighten it while leaning the upper body over and down, allowing the dumbbells to be pulled straight down.

Continue to inhale and focus on maintaining optimal posture as the leg is fully extended and the upper body is parallel with the floor and aligned straight with the leg.

Hold and balance at the bottom position; then slowly exhale, activate the core, pull the leg back up, and bring the torso to the starting position while relaxing the arms and maintaining proper posture.

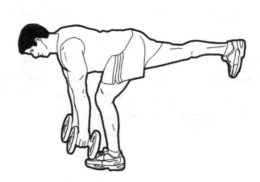

Cable Hip Abduction

Often, strengthening the body laterally in the frontal plane is overlooked in exercise routines. Typically, the gluteus medius and associated hip abductors are not strong muscles on the average person. Further, the symmetrical exercises most common for targeting hip and leg musculature, such as squats and leg presses, do very little for strengthening the hip abductors. Lunges and other standing, one-leg exercises will challenge these muscles but are often not found in a beginning program. These facts make this exercise a very valuable selection, particularly in base-building and early exercise programs. This standing position will train both sets of abductors simultaneously—one dynamically, the other statically—and provides better alignment and transference than the seated machine versions.

Alignment and Positioning

Strap one cable to the outside ankle and stand on a pad with the opposite foot straight ahead, aligned directly under the hip, and the knee slightly bent.

Position the movement leg slightly across the body and in front of the stationary leg with the opposite hand lightly on the bar for slight balance assistance.

Begin with the shoulders back, spine and head in posture, and draw a deep breath.

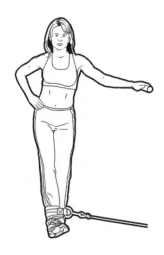

Motion and Stabilization

Slowly exhale; activate the core and pull the leg across and out from the body while maintaining proper posture and pelvic position.

Hold at the out position; then slowly inhale and allow the leg to be pulled back to the starting position while maintaining proper posture.

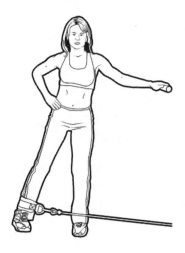

Cable Hip Adduction

Strengthening the body laterally in the frontal plane is one of the most overlooked components in many exercise routines. Typically, the adductors are not strong muscles on the average person; however, they are challenged as hip extensors in symmetrical exercises often performed for strengthening hip and leg musculature, such as squats and leg presses. These versatile muscles can also be challenged as hip flexors depending on the angle of pull to the resistance, so they will also get some work with various hip flexion exercises as well. However, more direct work such as this exercise may also be needed to achieve optimal balanced strengthening of the hip or stabilization of the pelvis. The standing position will train both sets of adductors simultaneously—one dynamically, the other statically—and has better transference than the seated machine versions.

Alignment and Positioning

Strap one cable to the inside ankle and stand on a pad with the opposite foot straight ahead, aligned directly under the hip, and the knee slightly bent.

Position the other leg about 45 degrees out from the body with the same side hand resting lightly on the bar for slight balance assistance.

Begin with the shoulders back, spine and head in posture, and draw a deep breath.

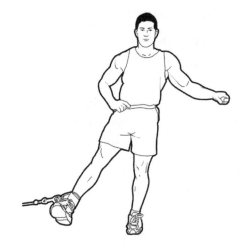

Motion and Stabilization

Slowly exhale; activate the core and pull the leg in and slightly across the body while maintaining proper posture and pelvic position.

Hold this position; then slowly inhale and allow the leg to be pulled back out to the starting position while maintaining proper posture.

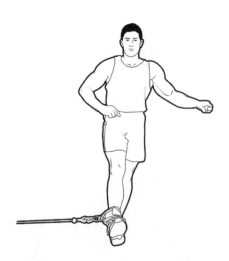

Body Weight Squat

This exercise is truly a functional movement that all walking people perform in some manner several times a day. Each descent into and rise from a chair, and each movement needed to bend and pick up any larger object directly in front of the body, is most often a squat movement. Although the exact foot positions, angle of body lean, and range of motion will vary in these everyday activities, the technique performed during the squat exercise teaches balance and body control that are highly transferable for these similar demands. Learning how to squat is also important for rehab from back, hip, knee, or even ankle injuries. Performing this movement without compensation is a must for the return to normal life.

Alignment and Positioning

Position the feet just outside shoulder width and angled out about 10–20 degrees.

Begin with the shoulders back, spine and head in posture, the knees and hips slightly bent, and the trunk in a slightly forward lean.

Exhale and activate the core.

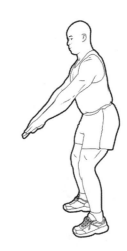

Motion and Stabilization

Slowly inhale; push the hips back, raise the arms, and allow the knees to bend naturally and the trunk to lean forward.

Lower the body until the crest of the pelvis presses against the top of the thigh or as far as possible while maintaining proper posture.

Hold; then slowly exhale, activate the core, and press the body back up to the starting position, relaxing the arms and maintaining proper posture.

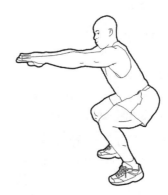

Balance Squat

This exercise is similar to the previous body weight squat but has additional balance demands. A balance board provides a specific tilting response reflex that is beneficial for certain goals. The long median plane fulcrum used in this demonstration is great for developing increased hip response and stability training and recruits more of the adductor muscles than a regular squat. A frontal plane fulcrum or smaller, rounded fulcrum, as well as utilizing stability disks, all will challenge the ankles more for reflex responses and stability. Choose the proper training tool for the desired effects and the appropriate goals.

Alignment and Positioning

Position the feet just outside shoulder width and angled out about 10–20 degrees.

Begin with the arms close to the body, and the spine and head in good posture.

Slightly bend the knees and hips, lean the trunk slightly forward, and then exhale and activate the core.

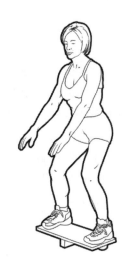

Motion and Stabilization

Slowly inhale; push the hips back; allow the knees to bend naturally and the trunk to lean forward.

Lower the body until the crest of the pelvis presses against the top of the thigh or as far as possible while maintaining proper posture.

Hold; then slowly exhale, activate the core, and press the body back up to the starting position while maintaining proper posture and letting the arms fall back to the starting position.

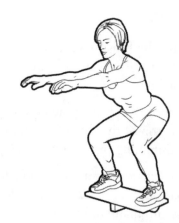

Dumbbell, Wide Squats

This exercise is similar to any squat movement. A wider stance is used to allow the dumbbell and arms to drop between the legs. This exercise targets the hip and knee extensors, but also works posterior trunk muscles as stabilizers and loads the squat in a manner very transferable to life demands. Most people must routinely perform this movement pattern to pick up a box, container, or other miscellaneous objects. Heavy loads are difficult to perform with this exercise, as the dumbbell will tend to protract the scapula, which in turn encourages flexion of the thoracic spine, reducing optimal posture. If heavier loads are desired, perhaps the barbell squat will be a better choice.

Alignment and Positioning

Position the feet well outside shoulder width and angled out about 30–40 degrees.

Begin by holding the dumbbell between the legs with the arms straight, and the spine and head in good posture.

Slightly bend the knees and hips, lean the trunk slightly forward; exhale and activate the core.

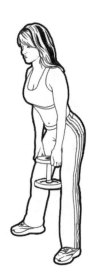

Motion and Stabilization

Slowly inhale; push the hips back; allow the knees to bend naturally and the trunk to lean forward.

Lower the body until the crest of the pelvis presses against the top of the thigh, or as far as possible while maintaining proper posture.

Hold; then slowly exhale, activate the core, and press the body and dumbbell back up to the starting position while maintaining proper posture.

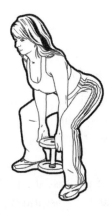

Dumbbell, Narrow Squats

This exercise is performed similar to any of the squat exercises only with a narrower stance to allow for the dumbbells and arms to drop comfortably outside the legs. This exercise begins with loading of the squat in a manner similar to certain demands of lifting suitcases and briefcases in life situations. Iso-lateral loading can also be done by simply using only one dumbbell, whenever desired. This exercise targets the hip and knee extensors and also works the posterior trunk muscles as stabilizers. Heavy loads are difficult to perform with this exercise, as the dumbbells will tend to protract the scapula, which in turn encourages flexion of the thoracic spine, reducing optimal posture. If heavier loads are desired, perhaps the barbell squat will be a better choice.

Alignment and Positioning

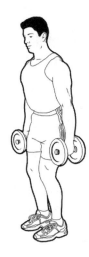

Position the feet just inside shoulder width and pointed straight ahead.

Begin by holding the dumbbells at the side, with the arms straight and the spine and head in good posture.

Slightly bend the knees and hips, lean the trunk slightly forward; exhale and activate the core.

Motion and Stabilization

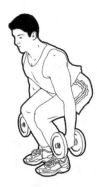

Slowly inhale; push the hips back; allow the knees to bend naturally and the trunk to lean forward.

Lower the body until the crest of the pelvis presses against the top of the thigh, or as far as possible while maintaining proper posture.

Hold at the bottom position; then slowly exhale, activate the core, and press the body and dumbbell back up to the starting position while maintaining proper posture.

Barbell Squats

This exercise is probably the best choice for maximally loading the squat movement. However, because in normal life situations we rarely place large loads on our backs and squat, this exercise is questionable as far as its direct transference. However, the capability for the back to stabilize while the legs move heavy loads might have other numerous indirect benefits. The added body strength and stability might increase the average person's ease and safety for daily lifting demands. However, athletes and exercise enthusiasts often use heavy barbell squats for hypertrophy goals or for increasing strength and one's potential for power.

Alignment and Positioning

Position the feet just outside shoulder width and angled out about 10–20 degrees.

Place the barbell just above the scapula with the hands placed comfortably on the bar and elbows pointed down.

Begin with the spine and head held in good posture, knees and hips bent, and the trunk leaned slightly forward.

Motion and Stabilization

Slowly inhale; push the hips back; allow the knees to bend naturally and the trunk to lean forward.

Lower the body until the crest of the pelvis presses against the top of the thigh, or as far as possible while maintaining proper posture.

Hold; then slowly exhale, activate the core, and press the body and barbell back up to the starting position while maintaining proper posture.

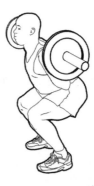

Barbell Dead-Lift

This exercise is similar to the traditional dead-lift, except with a modified starting position if needed to reduce lumbar disk compression and lower back strain. Dead-lifts are basically a squat movement challenging the hip and knee extensors with high stabilization demands for the spinal extensors. The primary difference from a barbell squat is that the dead-lift places the load inferior against the body's center of gravity. It is a more transferable exercise to life-lifting demands and is performed very similar to the dumbbell squat, except heavier loads can be used. Beginning each rep from a dead stop as presented is ideal for development of starting strength and acceleration strength, and more appropriate for certain goals.

Alignment and Positioning

Set the barbell at the appropriate height that allows to maintain natural lumbar curve and good posture at the bottom position.

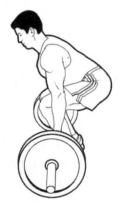

Position the feet just inside shoulder width and pointed straight ahead; grip the bar with a shoulder-width, alternate grip.

Begin in a squat position, hips and knees flexed, trunk leaned forward in good posture; draw a deep breath.

Motion and Stabilization

Slowly exhale; activate the core and press the body up, extending the hips and knees, pulling the shoulders back, pulling the bar up, and keeping it close to the legs.

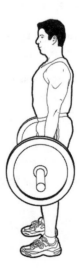

Stand completely up; hold the top position; then slowly inhale and squat, maintaining proper posture, lowering the bar and keeping it close to the legs until resting back on the rack. Stop; then repeat.

Machine, Seated Leg Press

This exercise targets and strengthens the hip and knee extensors. This might be ideal for achieving hypertrophy goals, dealing with prefatigue of the quadriceps and increase of lactic acid levels, or simply adding overall volume to a leg program. However, because the hip-and-knee action is performed in a seated and completely externally stabilized position, the carry-over strength and transference of this exercise are limited. Developing leg strength without proportional core, trunk, and hip stabilizer strength has questionable benefits for sports and life movements. Also, positioning of the spine and pelvis often is overlooked on such machines leading to S.I. joint stress and excessive lumbar disk compression. Be sure to maintain proper posture and foot placement at all times.

Alignment and Positioning

Position the back pad and feet in a manner that allows you to maintain an arch in the lower back and keeps the knees from passing too far over the toes at the bottom position.

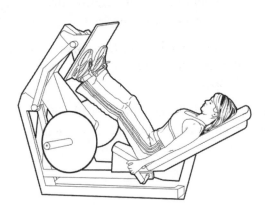

For a wide stance, position the feet just outside shoulder width and angled out about 20–30 degrees. For a narrow stance, feet should be no closer than hip width with feet positioned straight.

Begin with a slight bend in hips and knees, natural arch in the lower back, and the core activated.

Motion and Stabilization

Slowly inhale and allow the legs and platform to come down until the crest of the pelvis presses against the top of the thigh, or as far as possible while maintaining proper posture.

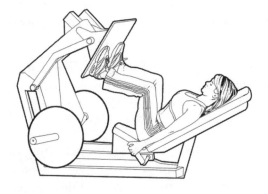

Hold; slowly exhale, activate the core, and press the legs and platform back up to the starting position while maintaining proper posture.

Body Weight, Stationary Lunge

This exercise is good to begin the strengthening of the lunge movement. Often, lunges are considered similar to a single leg squat, so they should be integrated into a program well after the squat has been mastered with additional loads. This movement prepares the body for stabilizing and pressing in an asymmetrical position that is sometimes required in certain sports—and in life. It also ensures more equal development of each leg with less possibility for compensation from the stronger side. Positioning of the trunk, hips, and ankles is critical for maximal safety and efficiency.

Alignment and Positioning

Position the legs in a lunge position that is long enough to provide for the desired range of motion.

Straighten the back leg and lean forward so that the trunk is in line with the back leg while maintaining proper posture.

Begin with a slight bend in the lead hip and knee, natural arch in the lower back, and the core activated.

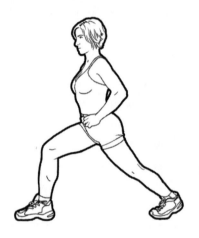

Motion and Stabilization

Slowly inhale and allow the trunk to come forward and down, until the crest of the pelvis presses against the top of the thigh, or as far as possible while maintaining proper posture.

Be sure to keep the forward knee aligned straight with the angle of the foot and avoid having it pass too far in front of the toes. Keep the trunk aligned with the back leg.

Hold; slowly start to exhale while activating the core. With the weight toward the heel, press the body up to the starting position while maintaining proper posture.

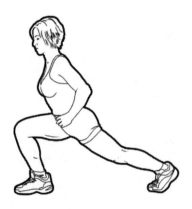

Dumbbell, Stationary Lunge

This exercise progresses the strengthening of the lunge movement. This movement prepares the body to stabilize and press in an asymmetrical position with added load. Maximal loads are difficult to use with this exercise as the heavier dumbbells will tend to protract the scapula, which in turn flexes the thoracic spine, diminishing optimal posture. To increase the challenge, you might want to either use a barbell or switch to a more dynamic lunge movement, such as a reverse lunge, depending on your goals. Positioning of the trunk, hips, and ankles is critical for maximal safety and efficiency.

Alignment and Positioning

Position the legs in a lunge position, long enough to provide for the desired range of motion.

Straighten the back leg and lean forward so that the trunk is in line with the back leg while maintaining proper posture.

Begin with the lead hip and knee bent, natural arch in the lower back, arms straight down, and the core activated.

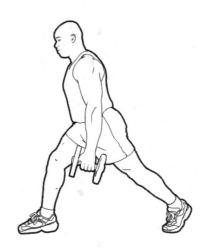

Motion and Stabilization

Slowly inhale and allow the trunk to come forward and down, until the crest of the pelvis presses against the top of the thigh, or as far as possible while maintaining proper posture.

Be sure to keep the forward knee aligned straight with the angle of the foot and avoid having it pass too far in front of the toes. Keep the trunk aligned with the back leg.

Hold; slowly start to exhale while activating the core. With the weight toward the heel, press the body up to the starting position while maintaining proper posture.

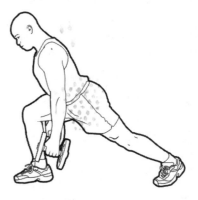

Body Weight, Reverse Lunge

This exercise progresses the lunge from a stationary exercise to a more dynamic movement. This exercise not only targets the hip and knee extensors of the forward leg; it challenges the hip abductors, as well as requires stabilization on one leg for most of the movement. This movement teaches the body balance and stabilization while on one leg, which is frequently needed during sports and often in life. Positioning of the trunk, hips, and ankles, and range of motion are all critical elements for maximal safety and efficiency. A crane technique is added to this exercise for greater balance challenges.

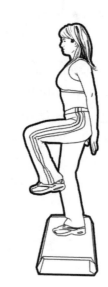

Alignment and Positioning

Stand with the weight on one leg and the other leg bent and held at a 90-degree angle in the crane position.

Position the trunk in good posture, activate the core, and begin with a slight bend in the knee and hip of the stationary leg.

Motion and Stabilization

Slowly inhale; while raising the arms out, step back and allow the torso to lean forward to a point where the crest of the pelvis touches the top of the thigh of the stationary leg, or as far as comfortable for desired range of motion.

Be sure to keep the forward knee aligned straight with the angle of the foot and avoid having it pass too far in front of the toes. Keep the trunk aligned with the back leg.

Hold; slowly start to exhale while activating the core; with the weight toward the heel, press the body up and pull the opposite leg back up to the starting position, while maintaining proper posture. Repeat or alternate legs.

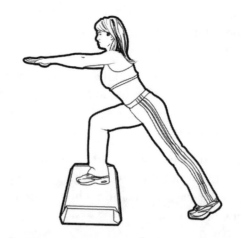

Dumbbell, Reverse Lunge

This exercise loads the lunge while performing a dynamic movement. It not only targets the hip and knee extensors of the forward leg, it challenges the hip abductors, as well, for balance and stabilization requirements. Maximal loads are difficult as the heavier dumbbells tend to protract the scapula and flex the thoracic spine, diminishing optimal posture. You can use steps to increase range of motion without stepping back as far, and to add increased deceleration demands. A crane technique is added for increased balance challenges.

Alignment and Positioning

Stand on a small step with the weight on one leg and other leg bent and held at a 90-degree angle in the crane position.

Position the trunk in good posture, activate the core, and begin with the arms and dumbbells straight down and a slight bend in the knee and hip of the stationary leg.

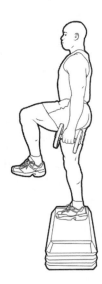

Motion and Stabilization

Slowly inhale and step back off the step and allow the torso to lean forward to a point where the crest of the pelvis touches the top of the thigh of the stance leg, or as far as comfortable for desired range of motion.

Be sure to keep the forward knee aligned straight with the angle of the foot and avoid having it pass too far in front of the toes. Keep the trunk aligned with the back leg.

Hold; slowly start to exhale while activating the core; with the weight toward the heel, press the trunk up and pull the opposite leg back up to the starting position while maintaining proper posture.

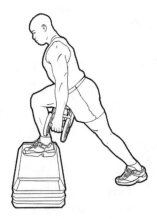

Traveling Lunge

This exercise begins training the lunge in a totally dynamic manner. This movement is difficult to perform with consistent technique as the entire body is in motion. This exercise will teach dynamic stabilization of the pelvis and trunk and requires high levels of balance. Mastering stationary and reverse lunges is helpful before proceeding to the traveling lunge as you will be very familiar with the proper positioning for the mid-point or bottom position of the exercise. Proper trunk, hip, and ankle positioning is critical throughout the movement for optimal safety and efficiency.

Alignment and Positioning

Stand with the weight on one leg and the toe of the other just touching the ground for balance.

Position the trunk in good posture, activate the core, and begin with a slight bend in the knee and hip of the stance leg.

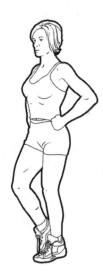

Motion and Stabilization

Slowly inhale; step forward and lean the trunk forward to a point where the crest of the pelvis touches the top of the thigh of the lead leg, or as far as comfortable for desired range of motion.

Be sure to keep the forward knee aligned straight with the angle of the foot, and avoid having it pass too far in front of the toes. Keep the trunk aligned with the back leg.

Hold; slowly exhale and activate the core; with the weight toward the heel, press the body forward and up to the starting position while maintaining proper posture. Repeat with the same leg or alternate.

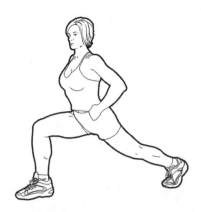

Dumbbell, Traveling Lunge

This exercise begins loading of the traveling lunge. Maximal loads are difficult as the heavier dumbbells tend to protract the scapula and flex the thoracic spine, diminishing optimal posture. This exercise teaches dynamic stabilization of the pelvis and trunk and requires high levels of balance. Mastering stationary and reverse lunges is helpful before proceeding to any traveling lunge as you will be very familiar with the proper positioning for the mid-point or bottom position of the exercise. Proper trunk, hip, and ankle positioning is critical throughout the movement for optimal safety and efficiency.

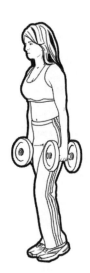

Alignment and Positioning

Stand with the weight on one leg and the toe of the other just touching the ground for balance.

Position the trunk in good posture, activate the core, and begin with a slight bend in the knee and hip of the stance leg.

Motion and Stabilization

Slowly inhale; step forward and lean the trunk forward to a point where the crest of the pelvis touches the top of the thigh of the lead leg, or as far as comfortable for desired range of motion.

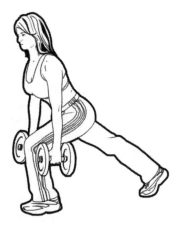

Be sure to keep the forward knee aligned straight with the angle of the foot and avoid having it pass too far in front of the toes. Keep the trunk aligned with the back leg.

Hold; slowly exhale, activate the core, and with the weight toward the heel, press the body forward and up to the starting position while maintaining proper posture. Repeat with the same leg or alternate.

Med Ball, Traveling Lunge (Side Load)

Using a med ball for added resistance makes different load placements more comfortable than using plates or dumbbells. You can place loads in front for a balanced anterior challenge, or to the side for an unbalanced lateral and stabilization challenge. For heavier posterior loads, a barbell probably would work the best. Choose the appropriate level and placement of loads to match the abilities and specific goals you presently possess. Only light to moderate loads are typically needed for any traveling lunge as maximum strength development is not the goal of this exercise.

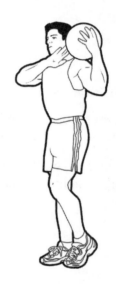

Alignment and Positioning

Stand with the weight on one leg and the toe of the other just touching the ground for balance.

Position the ball on the shoulder with the trunk in good posture. Activate the core and begin with a slight bend in the knee and hip of the stance leg.

Motion and Stabilization

Slowly inhale; step forward and lean the trunk forward to a point where the crest of the pelvis touches the top of the thigh of the lead leg, or as far as comfortable for desired range of motion.

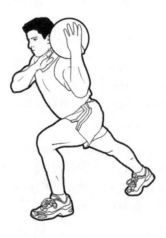

Be sure to keep the forward knee aligned straight with the angle of the foot and avoid having it pass too far in front of the toes. Keep the trunk aligned with the back leg.

Hold; slowly exhale, activate the core, and with the weight toward the heel, press the body forward and up to the starting position while maintaining proper posture. Repeat with the same leg or alternate.

Cable, Quad Extension

This exercise loads the extension movement of the knee targeting the quadriceps. However, the hip flexor and tibialis of the loaded leg, as well as the hip extensors and abductors of the stationary leg, will also be challenged as assistors and stabilizers. Core and trunk muscles will also work to stabilize the spine and pelvis. More or less stabilization from these muscles is required depending on the stability provided by the hands holding on to the machine. An active stretch of the gastrocs and hamstring muscles of the movement leg is also accomplished by flexing the hip and ankle while extending the knee.

Alignment and Positioning

Stand with the weight on one leg and the foot or ankle of the other leg in the strap, depending on the machine.

Pull the movement leg slightly up and in front of the stationary leg and position the trunk in good posture.

Draw a deep breath and begin with a slight bend in the knee and hip of the stance leg.

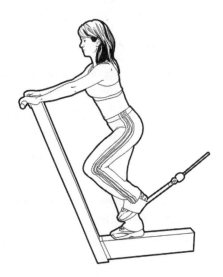

Motion and Stabilization

Slowly exhale; activate the core and pull the leg slightly forward as you extend the knee and pull back the toes.

Continue to pull the leg up and extend the knee until almost locked, causing a stretch on the hamstrings while maintaining posture and further activating the core.

Hold; slowly inhale and allow the leg to be pulled back to the starting position while maintaining posture.

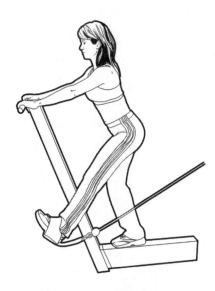

Machine, Quad Extension

This exercise loads and isolates the extension movement of the knees. This might be ideal for hypertrophy goals, prefatigue of the quadriceps, increase of lactic acid levels, or simply adding overall volume to a leg program. However, because you perform the knee action in a seated and completely externally stabilized position, the carry-over strength and transference of this exercise are limited. Developing leg strength without proportional core, trunk, and hip stabilizer strength has questionable benefits for sports and life movements. Also, be careful about the amount of resistance you use, as this machine creates a direct shearing force across the knees that is proportional to the amount of load.

Alignment and Positioning

Set the seat so that the knee joint is aligned with the axis and the pad is pressing against the shin.

Sit away from, or against, the back pad—depending on hamstring flexibility—so that a full extension of the knee is not quite possible when maintaining the natural arch in the lower back.

Position the trunk and pelvis in proper posture, begin with the knee flexed no more than 90 degrees and aligned with the toes, and then draw a deep breath.

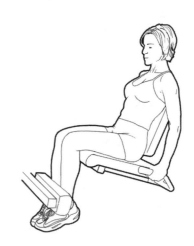

Motion and Stabilization

Slowly exhale; activate the core and pull the legs up and the toes back while maintaining posture.

Continue to pull the legs up until almost locked, causing a stretch on the hamstrings while maintaining posture and further activating the core.

Hold; slowly inhale and allow the legs to be pulled down to the starting position while maintaining posture.

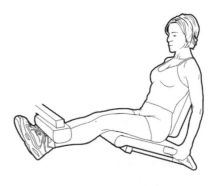

Cable, Ham Flexion

This exercise loads the flexion movement of the knee targeting the hamstrings. However, the hip extensors and gastrocs of the loaded leg, as well as the hip and knee extensors and abductors of the stationary leg, will also be challenged as assistors and stabilizers. Core and trunk muscles will also be worked to stabilize the spine and pelvis. More or less stabilization from these muscles is required depending on the level of stability provided by the hands holding on to the machine. An active stretch of the hip flexor muscles of the movement leg can also be accomplished with proper hip positioning and technique, providing another potential benefit for this exercise.

Alignment and Positioning

Stand with the weight on one leg and the foot or ankle of the other leg in the strap, depending on the machine.

Pull the movement leg slightly behind the stationary leg and position the trunk in good posture.

Draw a deep breath and begin with a slight bend in the knee and hip of the stance leg.

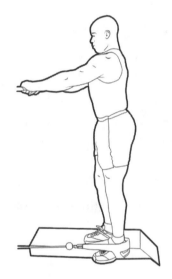

Motion and Stabilization

Slowly exhale; activate the core and pull the leg slightly back as you flex the knee and relax the foot.

Continue to pull the leg back and flex the knee to about 90 degrees, causing a slight stretch on the hip flexors while maintaining posture and further activating the core.

Hold; then slowly inhale and allow the leg to be pulled back to the starting position while maintaining posture.

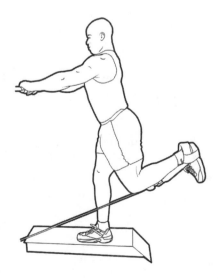

Machine, Ham Flexion

This exercise loads and isolates the flexion movement of the knees. This might be ideal for hypertrophy goals, isolated strengthening of the hamstrings, or simply adding overall volume to a leg program. Because knee extension is a resisted movement in squats, presses, and lunges, a certain amount of straight knee flexion may be needed for balanced strengthening. However, because you perform the knee action in a prone and completely externally stabilized position, the carry-over strength and transference of this exercise are limited. Developing leg strength without proportional core, trunk, and hip stabilizer strength has questionable benefits for sports and life movements.

Alignment and Positioning

Lay prone on a bench so that the knee joint is aligned with the axis and the pad is set below the gastrocs.

Position the trunk and neck in proper posture with the head off the pad, looking straight down, with the chin tucked.

Begin with the knees slightly bent, pelvis pressed against the pad, feet straight and relaxed, and draw a deep breath.

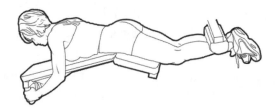

Motion and Stabilization

Slowly exhale; activate the core, press the pelvis tight into the pad while slightly raising the knees off the pad, and start to pull the legs up.

Continue to pull the legs up to about 90 degrees or as far as possible while maintaining posture and further activating the core.

Hold; slowly inhale and allow the legs to be pulled down to the starting position while maintaining posture.

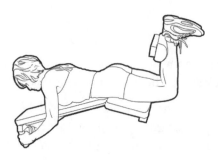

Dumbbell, One-Leg Calf Extension

This is one of the best and often overlooked exercise for training the ankle extensors. Balance is an integral part of this exercise. The ability of the ankle extensors to achieve strength levels that enable them to lift the entire body with additional loads is essential for anyone involved with activities that require take-offs and landings on one foot. This exercise is presented with slight balance assistance provided by the opposite arm but can be progressed to using no external anchor for increased balance challenges. You can also hold the dumbbell in the opposite arm to further offset center of gravity and increase balance demands.

Alignment and Positioning

Stand with the ball of one foot securely positioned on a step with the toes and entire leg rotated slightly out about 10 degrees for better balance, and the other leg bent.

Hold a dumbbell in the same side arm, place the opposite arm lightly on a wall or stable object for balance assistance, and then position the spine in good posture.

Begin with a slight bend in the stance leg and the heel slightly below the ball of the foot; then draw a deep breath.

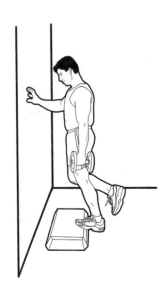

Motion and Stabilization

Slowly exhale; activate the core and extend the ankle, lifting the body up as far as possible while keeping the ankle from rolling out and the weight over the ball of the foot.

Hold; slowly inhale and allow the body to lower down to the starting position, maintaining proper posture and ankle positioning.

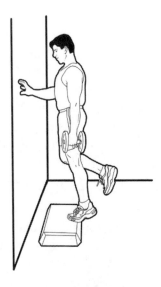

Machine Calf Extension

This exercise strengthens the ankle extensors. With the added balance and lever system of the machine, you can use heavier loads. This might be ideal for hypertrophy or isolated strengthening goals but might not transfer much to the demands placed on the ankle during dynamic movements under high forces. Because the gastrocs are two joint muscles prone to active insufficiency, it is not advised to attempt maximal depth with heavy loads. Try to avoid having the weight force more flexion of the ankles than you can actively create by pulling the toes up. This exercise can also be done with one leg at a time for isolateral strengthening of the ankles.

Alignment and Positioning

Stand with the balls of the feet securely positioned on a step with the toes and legs rotated slightly out about 10 degrees for better balance.

Pull the shoulders back and position the spine in good posture; then press the shoulders firmly up against the pads.

Begin with a slight bend in the knees and the heels slightly below the balls of the feet; then draw a deep breath.

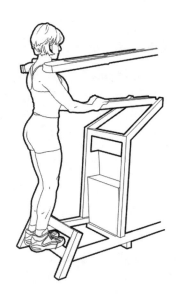

Motion and Stabilization

Slowly exhale, activate the core, and extend the ankles, lifting the body as far as possible while keeping the ankles from rolling out and the weight over the balls of the feet.

Hold; then slowly inhale and allow the body to lower to the starting position, while maintaining proper posture and ankle positioning.

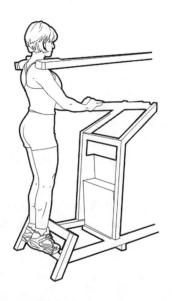

Machine, Bent-Leg Calf Extension

This exercise strengthens the ankle extensors and focuses primarily on the soleus. Targeting of this muscle might be ideal for hypertrophy or isolated strengthening goals, but might not transfer much to the demands placed on the ankle during dynamic movements under high forces. Because the gastrocs are two joint muscles, by bending the knee they are preshortened and become actively insufficient, leaving the soleus to carry most of the load. Try to avoid having the weight force more flexion of the ankles than you can actively create by pulling the toes up. This exercise can also be done with one leg at a time for iso-lateral strengthening of the ankles.

Alignment and Positioning

Sit with the balls of the feet securely positioned on the step with the toes and legs rotated slightly out about 10 degrees to better maintain ankle positioning.

Place the knees under the pads, pull the shoulders back, and position the spine in good posture.

Begin with the heels slightly below the balls of the feet; then draw a deep breath.

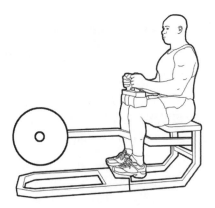

Motion and Stabilization

Slowly exhale; activate the core; and extend the ankles, lifting the knees and weight as high as possible while keeping the ankles from rolling out and the weight over the balls of the feet.

Hold; slowly inhale and allow the legs to lower to the starting position, maintaining proper posture and ankle positioning.

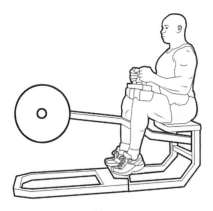

Machine Tib Flexion

This exercise strengthens the ankle flexors, primarily the tibialis anterior. As strengthening exercises for the ankle extensors are common in training programs, these important flexors of the ankle are most often overlooked. Maintaining a relatively balanced amount of strength around any joint is a key for its optimal performance and diminished potential for injury. This exercise can also serve as an active stretching exercise of the gastrocs and Achilles' tendon when done properly and with a full concentric range of motion.

Alignment and Positioning

Stand with the foot placed securely under the pad, with the ankle aligned with the axis of the machine.

Straighten and lock the knee of the working leg and position the foot parallel to the ground with the ankle extended about 40 degrees.

Stand in good posture while balancing on one leg and draw a deep breath.

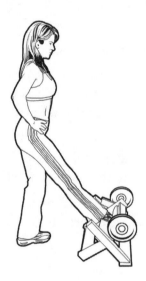

Motion and Stabilization

Slowly exhale; activate the core and flex the ankle, pulling the foot back as far as possible while keeping the toes relaxed and the knee locked.

Hold; slowly inhale and allow the foot to lower to the starting position, maintaining proper posture and ankle positioning.

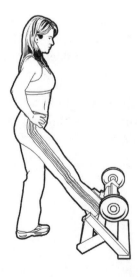

Iso-Kinetic Tib Flexion

This exercise strengthens the ankle flexors, primarily the tibialis anterior. Because strengthening exercises for the ankle extensors are common in training programs, these important flexors of the ankle are most often overlooked. As such is the case, equipment is often unavailable, but this exercise can easily be done with a partner. Maintaining a relative balanced amount of strength around any joint is a key for its optimal performance and decrease of potential injury.

Alignment and Positioning

Sit with the foot placed off the end of a bench so that the ankle is free to move.

Straighten and lock the knee of the working leg and position the foot straight with the ankle extended about 40 degrees.

Sit in good posture and draw a deep breath while your partner places a beginning resistance against the foot.

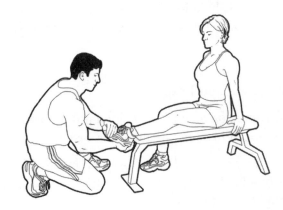

Motion and Stabilization

Slowly exhale; activate the core and flex the ankle, pulling the foot back as far as possible while keeping the toes relaxed and knee locked.

Your partner should apply a constant resistance at a level appropriate for achieving a full range of concentric motion.

Hold; slowly inhale and allow the foot to be pulled down to the starting position, maintaining proper posture and ankle positioning.

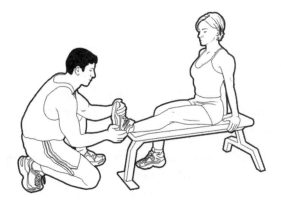

Upper Body Exercises

Dumbbell and Bench, Chest Press

This exercise targets strengthening of the chest and shoulder muscles, but will also incorporate the triceps as the elbow extensors as well. Dumbbells allow free movement of the hand and arm, resulting in a potential for increased shoulder adduction and increased shortening of the chest musculature than can be achieved with a barbell or most machines. Dumbbells also work each arm independently and therefore can be done with alternate movements, piston movements, or only one arm at a time. Choose the technique that is consistent with your present training phases and goals. A natural amount of scapula retraction is held for this exercise to protect the shoulder joint, as normal scapular-humeral rhythm is not possible while laying on a bench and pressing heavy weight.

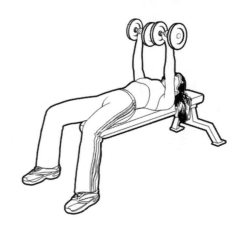

Alignment and Positioning

Lay supine on a bench with good posture and the feet braced firmly on the floor or a step.

Pull the shoulders slightly together and position the dumbbells perpendicular to the body, aligned straight over the shoulder.

Begin with the elbows pointed outward and slightly bent, wrists straight, and the core activated.

Motion and Stabilization

Slowly inhale; allow the arms to lower while pulling the elbows out and hands slightly away from each other.

Continue to lower the arms until the upper arm is almost parallel with the floor, with the hands slightly inside the elbows and maintaining good posture.

Hold; slowly exhale, contract the core, and press the arms and dumbbells back to the starting position, maintaining proper posture and scapula positioning.

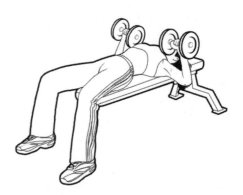

Dumbbell and Swiss Ball, One-Arm Chest Press

This exercise targets strengthening of the chest and shoulder muscles but will also place high demands on the trunk and core muscles. Because of a less stable base of support and unequal loading of the body, the obliques and associated trunk and hip muscles will be challenged to maintain proper posture against the resulting rotational forces. This might be ideal for developing more integrated actions of the trunk and upper extremity musculature, but would obviously not be the best choice for development of hypertrophy or maximal strength. This exercise can also be done with two arms using unequal loads for less rotational challenges or performed with alternate and piston movements for varied training effects. Choose the technique that is consistent with your present training phases and goals.

Alignment and Positioning

Lay supine on a Swiss ball with good posture and the feet braced firmly on the floor or a step.

Pull the shoulders slightly together and position the dumbbell perpendicular to the body, aligned straight over the shoulder.

Begin with the elbow pointed outward and slightly bent, wrist straight, and the core activated.

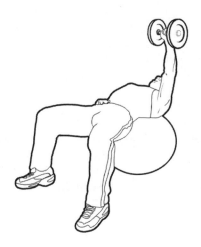

Motion and Stabilization

Slowly inhale and allow the arm to lower, keeping the hand slightly inside the elbow.

Continue to lower the arm until the upper arm is almost parallel with the floor, with the hand slightly inside the elbow, maintaining good posture.

Hold; slowly exhale, contract the core, and press the arm and dumbbell back to the starting position, maintaining proper posture.

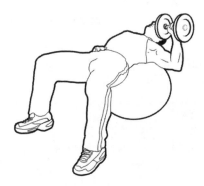

Barbell and Bench, Chest Press

This exercise targets the chest, shoulder, and triceps muscles. Pressing with a barbell forces a reciprocal, closed-chain action of the opposing arm that can be stressful to the shoulder joints once loaded, particularly if hand position is set incorrectly. Further risk is often applied due to the synergistic work of both arms enabling the lifter to move against heavier loads than when using individual dumbbells. It should also be noted that the strength obtained while lying on a bench will probably have little carryover for the pressing movements performed in sports and in life. In consideration of these facts, it is suggested that maximal loads not be used for this exercise. However, using maximal loads may be ideal for certain muscular endurance and hypertrophy goals.

Alignment and Positioning

Lay supine on a bench with good posture and the feet braced firmly on the floor or a step.

Pull the shoulder blades slightly together and place the hands on the bar so that a 90-degree angle is formed at the elbow when the bar is lowered.

Begin with good posture, bar over the chest, the elbows pointed out, wrists straight, and the core activated.

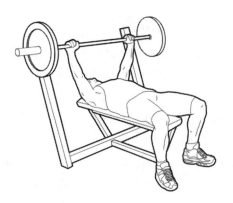

Motion and Stabilization

Slowly inhale; allow the arms and bar to lower while keeping the elbows under the bar and spine and pelvis set.

Continue to lower the bar until the arms are almost parallel with the floor, with the hands slightly inside the elbows while maintaining good posture.

Hold; slowly exhale, contract the core, and press the arms and barbell back to the starting position while maintaining proper posture and scapula positioning.

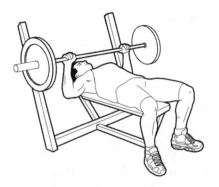

Squat Rack, Pushup

This exercise also targets the chest, shoulder, and triceps muscles. Performing pushups in this manner or off the floor forces the same reciprocal, closed-chain action that occurs with a barbell press. This can be stressful to the shoulder joints, particularly if hand position is not set properly. However, unlike with the barbell press, the strength obtained with this exercise has a much higher carryover to demands we encounter in sports and life situations. The pushup position also places load on the abdominal and hip flexors for stabilization requirements. Challenge can be decreased or increased by raising or lowering the angle of the body prior to beginning. Taking one foot from the ground also increases the challenge, particularly for the hip flexor of the support leg.

Alignment and Positioning

Position the barbell at the desired height for appropriate resistance and place the hands at a width that will form a 90-degree angle at the elbow when the body is lowered.

Align the body at an angle perpendicular to the arms with the balls of the feet firmly pressed against the floor.

Begin with good posture, elbows pointed out, wrists straight, and the core activated.

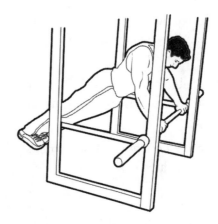

Motion and Stabilization

Slowly inhale; allow the body to lower while keeping the elbows pointed out and the spine and pelvis stabilized.

Continue to lower the body until an approximate 90-degree angle forms at the elbow.

Hold; slowly exhale, contract the core, and press the body back to the starting position, maintaining proper posture and scapula positioning.

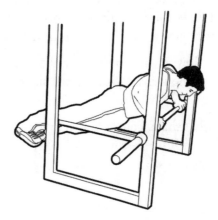

Cable One-Arm Decline Press (Lunge Position)

This exercise targets the mid and lower chest or sternal pecs, the anterior deltoids, and some triceps. However, pressing with one arm in the lunge position also integrates the same-side obliques, associated core and abdominal muscles, the contra-lateral hip flexors, and adductors. This synchronized sling of crossing trunk and lower body musculature is known collectively as the *anterior oblique subsystem*. Its designed action stabilizes the trunk and pelvis against anterior forces, but is also used for powerful rotational movements such as throwing, punching, or swinging bats and clubs. Strengthening the anterior oblique subsystem is a wise prerequisite for safe and efficient performance of any of these activities.

Alignment and Positioning

Stand in a lunge position with feet about shoulder width apart and the trunk leaned forward in good posture.

Position the cable handle down, perpendicular to the body and aligned straight with the shoulder and upper pulley.

Begin with the elbow pointed out, wrist straight, and the core activated.

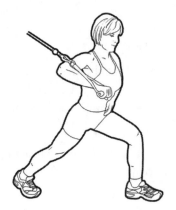

Motion and Stabilization

Slowly inhale; allowing the arm to be pulled out and up while keeping the hand slightly inside the elbow and avoiding any movement of the trunk.

Continue allowing the arm to be pulled back until the elbow is about even with the shoulder, and the hand is angled slightly in.

Hold; slowly exhale, contract the core, and press the arm back to the starting position while maintaining proper posture.

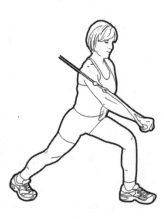

Dumbbell and Bench, Incline Press

This exercise targets strengthening of the upper chest or clavicular pectoralis muscles, and also incorporates the anterior deltoids and triceps. Dumbbells work each arm independently to allow for more movement of the shoulder and increased shortening of the chest musculature. You can perform this exercise with alternate movements, piston movements, or only one arm at a time. Choose the technique that is consistent with your present training phases and goals.

Note: A natural scapula retraction is held for this exercise to protect the shoulder joint, as normal scapular-humeral rhythm is not possible while lying on a bench and pressing heavy weight.

Alignment and Positioning

Lay supine on a bench angled anywhere between 30–60 degrees, with good posture and the feet braced firmly on the floor or a step.

Pull the shoulders slightly together and position the dumbbells perpendicular to the body, aligned straight over the shoulder.

Begin with the elbows pointed out and slightly bent, wrists straight, and the core activated.

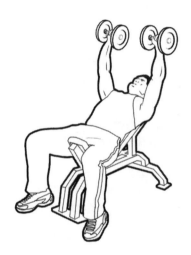

Motion and Stabilization

Slowly inhale; allow the arms to lower, pulling the elbows out and keeping hands slightly away from each other.

Continue to lower the arms until the arms are almost parallel with the floor, with the hands slightly inside the elbows while maintaining good posture.

Hold; slowly exhale, contract the core, and press the arms and dumbbells back to the starting position, maintaining proper posture and scapula positioning.

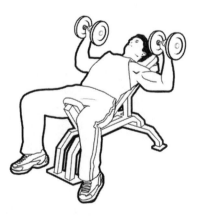

Dumbbell and Swiss Ball, One-Arm Incline Press

This exercise targets the upper chest or clavicular pectoralis, anterior deltoids, and triceps muscles. This exercise also challenges the trunk and core muscles. Because of working on a less stable base of support and unequal loading of the body, there is a high demand on the obliques and associated trunk and hip muscles to maintain proper posture against the resulting rotational forces. Exercises done on the ball also require more neck flexor strength, as the head is not supported throughout the exercise. You can also do this exercise with two arms using unequal loads for less rotational challenges. Alternate arm movements and piston movements can also be used for varied training effects.

Alignment and Positioning

Lie at a 30- to 60-degree angle on a Swiss ball with good posture and the feet braced firmly on the floor or a step.

Pull the shoulders slightly together and position the dumbbell perpendicular to the body, aligned straight over the shoulder.

Begin with the elbow pointed out and slightly bent, wrist straight, and the core activated.

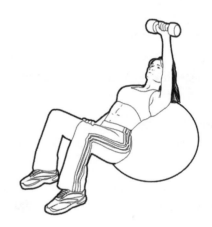

Motion and Stabilization

Slowly inhale; allow the arm to lower while keeping the hand slightly inside the elbow and avoiding any rotation of the trunk.

Continue to lower until the upper arm is almost parallel with the floor, with the hand slightly inside the elbow while maintaining good posture.

Hold; slowly exhale, contract the core, and press the arm and dumbbell back to the starting position while maintaining proper posture.

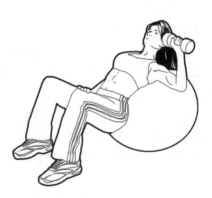

Dumbbell, Delt Press (Lunge Position)

This exercise targets the anterior deltoids, but also works some upper chest and triceps. This exercise also requires an upward rotation of the scapula, which subsequently will work the trapezius muscles as well. The core, trunk, hip, and leg muscles will all be challenged, as well, to stabilize the body during the press. Lunge positions, as presented here, place more load on the glute and quads of the lead leg, and provide less stability in the frontal plane, requiring more work of the hip abductors. You can add balancing challenges by performing this exercise on an unstable surface or simply standing on one leg. You can also perform this exercise with offset loads, alternate movements, and piston movements for varied training effects.

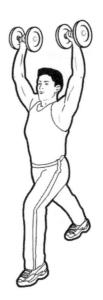

Alignment and Positioning

Stand in a lunge position with feet about shoulder width apart and more weight placed on the forward leg.

Begin with the dumbbells overhead and perpendicular to the body, aligned straight over the shoulder, with the trunk held in good posture.

Begin with the elbows pointed out and slightly bent, wrist straight, and the core activated.

Motion and Stabilization

Inhale and allow the arms to lower, keeping the hands slightly inside the elbow and avoiding any movement of the trunk.

Continue to lower the arms until they are just parallel to the floor, keeping the hands slightly inside the elbow and maintaining good posture.

Hold; slowly exhale, contract the core, and press the dumbbells back to the starting position while maintaining proper posture.

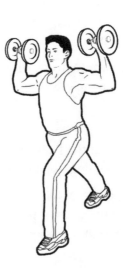

Dumbbell, One-Arm and One-Leg, Delt Press

This exercise works the anterior deltoid, trapezius, and some upper chest muscles and triceps; it demands high levels of involvement for the core, trunk, and hip muscles to stabilize the body. Performing upper extremity exercises while balancing on one leg might have more carryover to certain sports and life activities than most would think. The more often we carry loads up or down stairs; step on or off ladders; or lift, press, or pull while on one leg—for any reason—the more valuable this type of exercise is to our programs. You can also perform this exercise using the opposite arm of the support leg for greater balance challenge.

Alignment and Positioning

Stand on one leg with the other foot off the ground and position the trunk in good posture.

Begin with the same-side dumbbell overhead, perpendicular to the body, and aligned straight over the shoulder.

Point the elbow out, slightly bent, wrist straight, and the core activated.

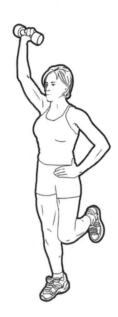

Motion and Stabilization

Inhale and allow the arm to lower while keeping the hand slightly inside the elbow and avoiding any movement of the trunk.

Continue to lower until the upper arm is almost parallel to the floor, with the hand slightly inside the elbow while maintaining good posture.

Hold; slowly exhale, contract the core, and press the dumbbell back to the starting position while maintaining proper posture.

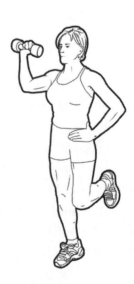

Barbell Lat Row

This exercise targets the lats, scapular retractors, rear deltoids, and biceps. In addition, the vertical pull of the resistance against the trunk challenges the spinal erectors and hip extensors to provide trunk and pelvic stability. Performing rowing exercises with free weights requires a high level of hamstring flexibility to align the body in opposition to gravity and still maintain natural lumbar curvature. Depending on training goals, using cable pulley systems or rowing machines might be a better option for targeting this movement and muscle groups until you achieve appropriate hamstring flexibility and lumbar stability.

Alignment and Positioning

Stand with the legs set just outside shoulder width and grasp the bar with an underhand grip exactly shoulder width apart.

Draw a deep breath, flex over at the hip, and bend the knees to allow for a natural arch to be set in the lower spine.

Begin with the arms straight, hands slightly in front of shoulders, scapula slightly protracted, and the spine in good posture.

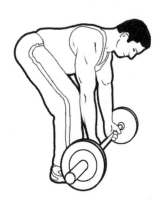

Motion and Stabilization

Slowly begin to exhale; activate the core and pull the shoulder blades together while pulling the arms back and up.

Continue to retract the scapula, activate the core, and pull the arms up and barbell toward the umbilicus until the upper arm is about parallel to the body while maintaining posture.

Hold; slowly inhale and allow the arms and scapula to be pulled back to the starting position while maintaining proper posture.

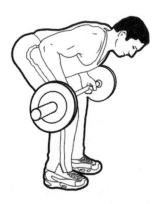

Dumbbell One-Arm Lat Row

This exercise targets the lats, scapular retractors, rear deltoids, and biceps. In addition, the vertical pull of the resistance against the trunk challenges the spinal erectors and hip extensors to provide trunk and pelvic stability. Using only one arm unequally loads the body and further challenges trunk and oblique muscles to stabilize against rotation of the spine. You can perform this exercise with a brace and in a symmetrical stance as presented here, or without a brace and in a lunge position depending on your goals. Hamstring flexibility must be appropriate to align against gravity and allow for proper lumbar curvature.

Alignment and Positioning

Stand with the legs aligned just inside shoulder width and hold a dumbbell with one hand.

Brace the other arm against the back of a bench, draw a deep breath, flex over at the hip, and bend the knees to set a natural arch in the lower spine.

Begin with the arm straight, hand slightly in front of shoulder, scapula slightly protracted, and the spine in good posture.

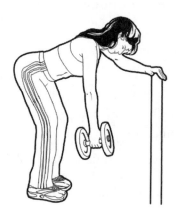

Motion and Stabilization

Slowly begin to exhale; activate the core and pull the shoulder blades together while pulling the arm back and up.

Continue to retract the scapula, activate the core, and pull the arm up and dumbbell toward the umbilicus until the upper arm is almost parallel to the body, while maintaining posture.

Hold; then slowly inhale and allow the arm and scapula to be pulled back to the starting position while maintaining proper posture.

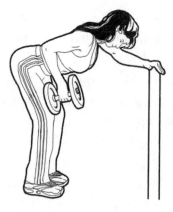

Cable, Seated Lat Row

This exercise targets the lats, scapular retractors, rear deltoids, and biceps. In addition, the perpendicular pull of the resistance against the trunk challenges the spinal erectors and associated postural muscles for trunk stability. Rowing exercises are pulling movements performed in the median plane, which allows for maximal shortening of the lats and should incorporate a natural scapular humeral rhythm that trains the scapular retractors and depressors. Maintaining proper posture is imperative for proper scapular movement and reduction of compressive forces on the lumbar disks.

Alignment and Positioning

Sit with the legs spread to allow for arm movement, and knees bent to allow for a natural arch in the lower spine.

Begin with the arms straight, scapula slightly protracted, and the spine in good posture; then draw a deep breath.

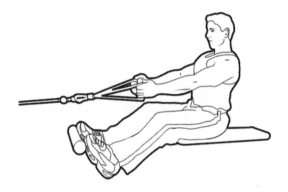

Motion and Stabilization

Slowly begin to exhale; activate the core and pull the shoulder blades together while pulling the arms down and back.

Continue to retract the scapula, activate the core, and pull the arms back until the elbow is aligned with the shoulder, or as far as possible while maintaining proper posture.

Hold; then slowly inhale and allow the arms and scapula to be pulled back to the starting position while maintaining proper posture.

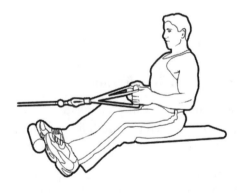

Cable, Overhead Lat Row

This exercise targets the lats, scapular retractors, rear deltoids, and biceps. The overhead angle allows for a much higher degree of resisted shoulder movement than the typical seated machines. Also, the standing position is more difficult to stabilize, as there is a drastic elevation of the body's center of gravity compared to a seated version. Training on the feet might be more transferable to most sports or life applications, but maximal loads are difficult to move in the standing position. If desired, this exercise can be performed seated or kneeling, to more easily apply heavier loads and increase the resisted range of motion. This may be more appropriate positioning for certain goals and training phases.

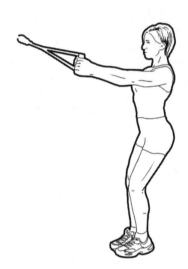

Alignment and Positioning

Grasp the handles; then step back from the pulley with the legs about shoulder-width apart.

Begin with the arms straight, scapula slightly protracted, and the weight more to the heels.

Position the spine in good posture; then draw a deep breath.

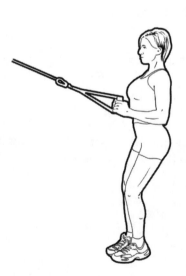

Motion and Stabilization

Slowly begin to exhale; activate the core and pull the shoulder blades together while pulling the arms down and back.

Continue to retract the scapula, activate the core, and pull the arms back until the elbow is aligned with the shoulder or as far as possible while maintaining proper posture.

Hold; then slowly inhale and allow the arms and scapula to be pulled back to the starting position while maintaining proper posture.

Cable, One-Arm Low Lat Row (Lunge Position)

This exercise targets the lats, scapular retractors, rear deltoids, biceps, and the postural muscles of the back and hip as well. Pulling with one arm in the lunge position activates more use of the thoraco-lumbar fascia, which integrates the lats with the contra-lateral glutes, and associated hip extensors and abductors. This synchronized sling of crossing trunk and lower body musculature is known collectively as the *posterior oblique subsystem*. Its designed functions are to stabilize the trunk and pelvis, propel the body during gait, and decelerate the body during powerful rotational movements such as throwing, punching, or swinging bats and clubs. Strengthening this system should assist in performance of these activities.

Alignment and Positioning

Grasp the handle; then step back from the pulley into a lunge position with the opposite leg forward and legs about shoulder width apart.

Begin with the arm aligned with the cable, scapula slightly protracted, and the weight mostly on the lead leg.

Position the spine in good posture; then draw a deep breath.

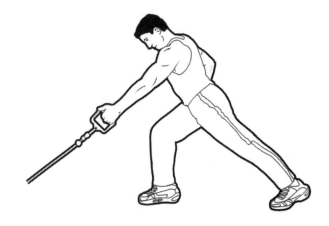

Motion and Stabilization

Slowly begin to exhale; activate the core and pull the shoulder blades together while pulling the arm back and up.

Continue to retract the scapula, activate the core, and pull the arm up and hand toward the lower sternum until the upper arm is almost parallel to the body.

Hold; then slowly inhale and allow the arm and scapula to be pulled back to the starting position while maintaining proper posture.

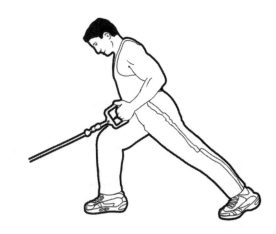

Cable, Seated Lat Pulldown

This exercise works the lats, but focuses more on training the rhomboids and associated scapular downward rotators and depressors. Pulling movements in the frontal plane require a more difficult scapular-humeral rhythm than the previous rowing movements that occur in the median plane. This scapular-humeral rhythm is critical for safe and efficient movements in this plane and is dependent on the ability to obtain proper posture of the thoracic spine. Therefore, you might need to introduce rowing movements into a program before adding pulling movements to develop the postural muscles that stabilize the spine and allow for safe execution of frontal plane exercises.

Alignment and Positioning

Sit with the knees braced just under the pad and lean slightly back from the hip so that the bar can pass in front of the face.

Set a natural arch in the lower spine and begin with the arms straight, elbows out, and the scapula elevated.

Position the spine in good posture with the chest up and draw a deep breath.

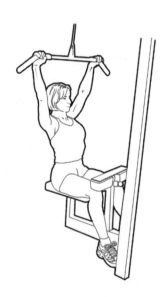

Motion and Stabilization

Slowly begin to exhale; activate the core and pull the shoulder blades down while pulling the elbows out and the bar down toward the clavicle.

Continue to depress the scapula, activate the core, lift the chest, and pull the arms down as far as possible while keeping the elbows slightly behind the hands.

Hold; then slowly inhale and allow the arms and scapula to be pulled back to the starting position while maintaining proper posture.

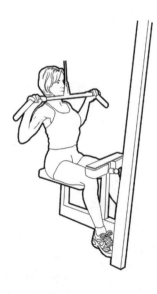

Machine, Lat Pull-Up

This exercise works the lats, but focuses more on training the rhomboids and associated scapular downward rotators and depressors. Although similar to the pull-down, the pull-up places slightly different demands on the shoulder and elbow musculature and is more transferable to the pulling movements we encounter outside the gym. Pull-ups are a great exercise to assess one's relative strength against his or her body weight and are very difficult for most people to perform without assistance. Scapular depressors are typically weak and the first to fail during this exercise—well before the ability to complete a pull-up. Proper technique is imperative to develop these muscles.

Alignment and Positioning

Grasp the bar well outside the shoulders so that a 90-degree angle forms at the elbow as you pull up.

Begin on the support bar with the arms straight, elbows slightly bent and pointed out, and the scapula elevated.

Position the spine in good posture with the chest up and draw a deep breath.

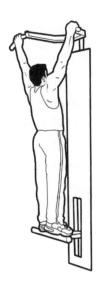

Motion and Stabilization

Slowly begin to exhale; activate the core and pull the shoulder blades down while pulling the elbows out and the body straight up without leaning.

Continue to depress the scapula, activate the core, lift the chest, and pull the body up as far as possible, keeping the body straight.

Hold; then slowly inhale and allow the body to be pulled back down and scapula to elevate back to the starting position while maintaining proper posture.

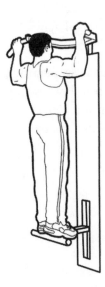

Dumbbell Rear Delt Row

This exercise targets the rear deltoids, scapular retractors, shoulder external rotators, and biceps. In addition, the vertical pull of the resistance directly challenges the spinal erectors and hip extensors for trunk and pelvic stability. Although free weight lifting performed on the feet will probably have more transference to sport-specific needs and life circumstances, these rowing exercises require a high level of hamstring flexibility to align the body properly against gravity. Depending on training goals, using cable pulley systems or rowing machines might be a better option until you achieve appropriate hamstring flexibility and lumbar stability.

Alignment and Positioning

Stand with the legs set just outside shoulder width with the feet angled 20–30 degrees.

Draw a deep breath; then flex over at the hip and bend the knees to allow for a natural arch in the lower spine.

Begin with the arms straight down from the shoulders with the elbows pointed out, scapula slightly protracted, and the spine in good posture.

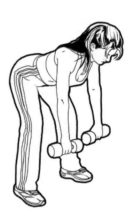

Motion and Stabilization

Slowly begin to exhale; activate the core and pull the shoulder blades together while pulling the arms out and up.

Continue to retract the scapula; activate the core and pull the arms up and out with the hands just inside the elbows until the arms are almost parallel to the floor, maintaining posture.

Hold; then slowly inhale and allow the arms and scapula to be pulled back to the starting position while maintaining proper posture.

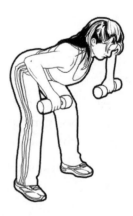

Cable, Overhead Rear Delt Row (Lunge Position)

This exercise targets the rear deltoids, but also works the scapular retractors, shoulder external rotators, and biceps. The overhead, standing position is more difficult to stabilize, because there is a drastic elevation of the body's center of gravity compared to a seated version. Training on the feet might be more transferable toward most sport-specific needs or for life applications, but maximal loads are difficult to move in the standing position. You can perform this exercise in seated or kneeling positions to more easily apply heavier loads for certain training phases and goals.

Alignment and Positioning

Grasp the handles; then step back from the pulley into a lunge position with the legs about shoulder width apart.

Begin with the arms straight with the cable and elbows pointed out, scapula slightly protracted, and more weight over the back leg.

Position the spine in good posture and draw a deep breath.

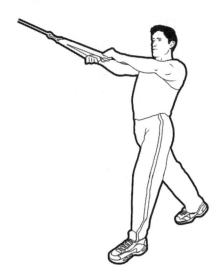

Motion and Stabilization

Slowly begin to exhale; activate the core and pull the shoulder blades together while pulling the arms out and back.

Continue to retract the scapula, activate the core, and pull the arms back and hands apart as far as possible.

Hold; then slowly inhale and allow the arms and scapula to be pulled back to the starting position while maintaining proper posture.

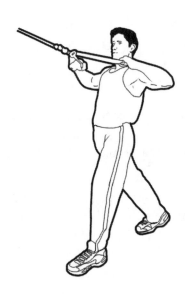

Cable, One-Arm Low Rear Delt Row (Lunge Position)

This exercise targets the rear deltoids, but also works the scapula retractors, shoulder external rotators, and biceps. Pulling from a low position with one arm unequally loads the body and requires high levels of trunk and hip extensor demand for stabilization against the downward rotational forces. The lunge position further loads the gluteus of the lead leg, associated hip extensors, and hip abductors as compared to a symmetrical stance. Pulling in lunge positions also activates the thoraco-lumbar fascia, and stimulates the entire posterior-oblique subsystem. This subsystem is designed to assist with stabilization of the trunk and pelvis, propels the body during gait, and decelerates the body and limbs during powerful rotational movements.

Alignment and Positioning

Grasp the handle; then step back from the pulley into a lunge position with the opposite leg forward and legs about shoulder width apart.

Begin with the arm aligned with the cable, elbow pointed out, scapula slightly protracted, and the weight mostly on the lead leg.

Position the spine in good posture and then draw a deep breath.

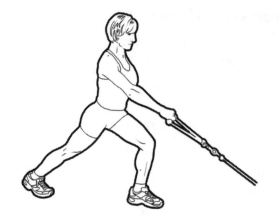

Motion and Stabilization

Slowly begin to exhale; activate the core and pull the shoulder blades together while pulling the arm out and up.

Continue to retract the scapula, activate the core, and pull the arm up and hand out, keeping the arms horizontal to the body and hand just inside the elbow.

Hold; then slowly inhale and allow the arm and scapula to be pulled back to the starting position while maintaining proper posture.

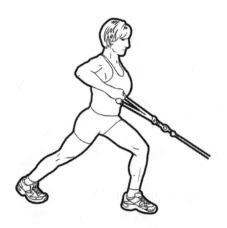

Barbell Scapular Elevation (Shrug)

This exercise targets the scapula elevators and can strengthen upper back and neck musculature in preparation for the initial movement of certain power training exercises or Olympic lifts, such as the power-clean, hang-clean, or snatch. The technique presented contains important modifications to the traditional shrug movement. The trunk is positioned in a forward lean at the hip to align for a direction of pull that utilizes more scapular retractors. This positioning, plus using a wider grip on the bar, provides for increased upward rotation of the scapula and helps to recruit more upper trapezius muscle. Also, this alignment and technique pull the shoulders behind the head, which decreases involvement of the levator scapula and reduces cervical disk compression.

Alignment and Positioning

Stand in good posture with the feet directly under the hips and grasp the bar with a wide overhand grip.

Push the hips back and flex over at the hips, creating a forward lean of the trunk with the knees slightly bent.

Position the spine in good posture and begin with the arms hanging straight down, bar against the thighs; then draw a deep breath.

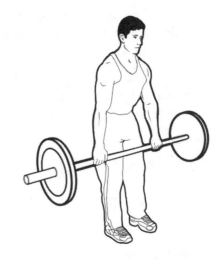

Motion and Stabilization

Slowly begin to exhale; activate the core and pull the shoulder blades up and together while keeping the arms relaxed.

Continue to elevate the scapula and activate the core, keeping good posture in the spine.

Hold; then slowly inhale and allow the arms and scapula to be pulled back to starting position while maintaining proper posture.

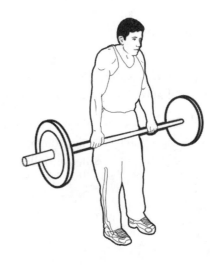

Dumbbell, Shoulder External Rotation

This exercise is designed to isolate and strengthen the rotator cuff muscles, particularly the infraspinatus and teres minor. The arm is stabilized in a slightly abducted position for better joint surface contact with the elbow held at 90 degrees to ensure a more isolated shoulder movement and targeting of the external rotators. This exercise obviously does not directly transfer to the integrated demands of the rotator cuff muscles needed for sport-specific movements or life activities. However, it might be ideal for beginning training of these muscles or for initial stages of rehabilitation goals.

Alignment and Positioning

Lie on your side in good posture with the hips and knees bent comfortably and the head supported by the bottom arm, as shown.

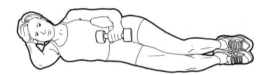

Place the elbow of the top arm on a folded towel to abduct the arm about 10–30 degrees, with the elbow bent at 90 degrees.

Stabilize the spine and shoulders in good posture, and begin with the arm rotated down; then draw a deep breath.

Motion and Stabilization

Exhale; activate the core and rotate the shoulder, pulling the lower arm and dumbbell up while keeping the wrist straight.

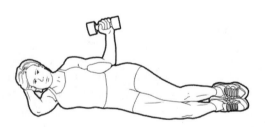

Continue to rotate the shoulder and pull the arm up as far as possible, keeping the elbow pressed against the towel and maintaining good posture.

Hold; then slowly inhale and allow the arm and dumbbell to be pulled back to the starting point while maintaining proper posture and elbow positioning.

Dumbbell, Shoulder Internal Rotation

This exercise is designed to isolate and strengthen the rotator cuff muscles, particularly the subscapalaris. The arm is stabilized in an abducted position for better joint surface contact, with the elbow held at 90 degrees to ensure a more isolated shoulder movement and targeting of the internal rotators. This exercise obviously does not directly transfer to the integrated demands of the rotator cuff muscles needed for sport-specific movements or life activities. However, it might be ideal for beginning training of these muscles or for initial stages of rehabilitation goals.

Alignment and Positioning

Lie on your side in good posture with the hips and knees bent comfortably and the head held in a neutral position.

Position the bottom arm with the shoulder flexed 70–80 degrees and elbow bent 90 degrees.

Stabilize the spine and shoulders in good posture and begin with the arm rotated down; then draw a deep breath.

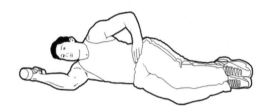

Motion and Stabilization

Exhale; activate the core and rotate the shoulder, pulling the lower arm and dumbbell up while keeping the wrist straight.

Continue to rotate the shoulder and pull the arm up until almost straight up, keeping the elbow pressed against the floor and maintaining good posture.

Hold; slowly inhale and allow the arm and dumbbell to be pulled back to the starting point while maintaining proper posture and elbow positioning.

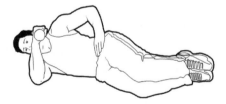

Cable, Shoulder Horizontal External Rotation

This exercise is designed for strengthening of the shoulder and rotator cuff muscles, particularly the infraspinatus and teres minor. The arm is stabilized slightly below 90 degrees of abduction for increased stabilization demand from the deltoid musculature during the rotational movement. Hold the elbow at 90 degrees and isolate the movement to ensure specific targeting of the external rotators. By being on the feet and increasing the involvement of the deltoids, you move toward the integrated demands of the rotator cuff, which you will need for sport-specific movements and life activities. You can use different shoulder angles as desired.

Alignment and Positioning

Stand in a lunge position and hold the lower cable handle with the arm abducted just below 90 degrees.

Position the elbow at 90 degrees and internally rotate the shoulder until the cable handle and forearm are in line with the lower pulley.

Stabilize the spine and shoulders in good posture; then draw a deep breath.

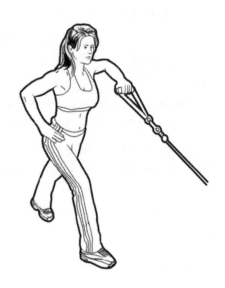

Motion and Stabilization

Exhale; activate the core and rotate the shoulder, pulling the lower arm and cable handle up while keeping the upper arm and wrist straight.

Continue to rotate the shoulder and pull the lower arm up as far as possible, keeping good posture and the upper arm just below parallel to the floor.

Hold; then slowly inhale and allow the arm and cable handle to be pulled back to the starting point while maintaining proper posture and elbow positioning.

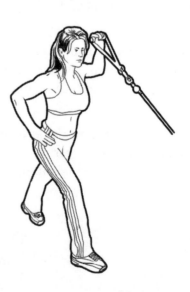

Cable, Shoulder Horizontal Internal Rotation

This exercise is designed to strengthen the shoulder and rotator cuff muscles, particularly the subscapalaris. The arm is stabilized slightly below 90 degrees of abduction for increased stabilization demand from the deltoid musculature during the rotational movement. Hold the elbow at 90 degrees and isolate the movement to ensure specific targeting of the external rotators. Being on the feet and working the deltoids in this manner helps begin to prepare you for the integrated demands of the rotator cuff, which you will need for sport-specific movements and life activities. You can use different shoulder angles as desired.

Alignment and Positioning

Stand in a lunge position and hold the upper cable handle with the arm abducted just below 90 degrees.

Position the elbow at 90 degrees and externally rotate the shoulder up as far as possible while keeping the upper arm about level.

Stabilize the spine and shoulders in good posture; draw a deep breath.

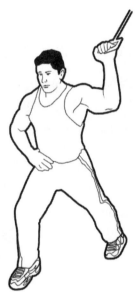

Motion and Stabilization

Exhale; activate the core and rotate the shoulder, pulling the lower arm and cable handle forward and down and keeping the upper arm and wrist straight.

Continue to rotate the shoulder and pull the arm down until the forearm is in line with the pulley, keeping the upper arm just below parallel to the floor.

Hold; then slowly inhale and allow the arm and cable handle to be pulled back to the starting point while maintaining proper posture and elbow positioning.

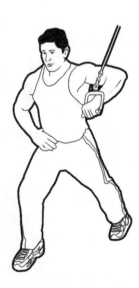

Cable, Shoulder-Integrated External Rotation

This exercise is designed to strengthen the shoulder and rotator cuff muscles, particularly the infraspinatus and teres minor. This movement trains the external rotators in a more integrated manner with involvement of deltoid and scapular muscles. This exercise is ideal for more advanced rotator cuff training and final stages of rehabilitation, and better prepares the rotator cuff and shoulder girdle for the integrated demands that will be needed for sport-specific movements and life activities. You can use different shoulder angles as desired.

Alignment and Positioning

With one arm, grasp the opposite-side, lower cable handle lengthwise, and then stand in good posture.

Position the arm across the body about 10–30 degrees. Internally rotate the shoulder so thumb is down and elbow is pointed forward and slightly bent.

Begin with the scapula slightly protracted, spine in good posture, and draw a deep breath.

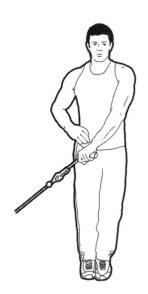

Motion and Stabilization

Slowly begin to exhale; activate the core and pull the arm across the body and up while externally rotating the shoulder and twisting the thumb up.

Continue to rotate the shoulder and pull the arm up as far as possible, keeping good posture and the elbow slightly bent.

Hold; then slowly inhale and allow the arm and cable handle to be pulled back to the starting point while maintaining proper posture and elbow positioning.

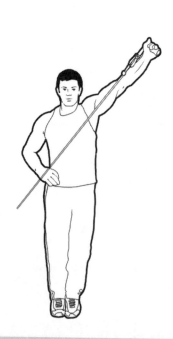

Cable, Shoulder-Integrated Internal Rotation

This exercise is designed for strengthening of the shoulder and rotator cuff muscles, particularly the subscapalaris. This movement trains the internal rotators to integrate the deltoid, scapular, and pectoralis muscles. It is ideal for more advanced rotator cuff training and final stages of rehabilitation and prepares the rotator cuff and shoulder girdle for the integrated demands of sport-specific movements and life activities. You can use different shoulder angles as desired.

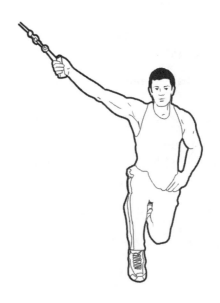

Alignment and Positioning

With one arm, grasp the opposite-side, upper cable handle lengthwise, and then stand or kneel in good posture.

Position the arm out and above the body abducted about 140–160 degrees. Externally rotate the shoulder so the thumb is up and the elbow is pointed out and slightly bent.

Begin with the scapula fully retracted and the spine in good posture; draw a deep breath.

Motion and Stabilization

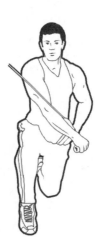

Slowly begin to exhale; activate the core and pull the arm out, down, and across the body while internally rotating the shoulder and twisting the thumb down.

Continue to rotate the shoulder and pull the arm down and slightly across the body, keeping good posture and the elbow slightly bent.

Hold; then slowly inhale and allow the arm and cable handle to be pulled back to the starting point while maintaining proper posture and elbow positioning.

Dumbbell and Swiss Ball, Triceps Extension

This exercise targets the triceps muscle group. The flexed shoulder position required for this exercise prelengthens the long-head triceps, keeping them active throughout the range of motion. Performing this exercise with dumbbells allows the wrists to remain in a neutral position and challenges each arm independently, demanding more from shoulder and rotator cuff muscles for stabilization. Alternately, you can do piston and single-arm movements with dumbbells. Using the Swiss ball will also require more core, trunk, neck, and hip muscle activation for balance and stabilization demands.

Alignment and Positioning

Lay on a Swiss ball at approximately a 45-degree angle, and hold a set of dumbbells parallel to the body, aligned straight above the shoulders.

Externally rotate the shoulders so that the elbow is pointing forward with a slight bend and the wrists are in neutral.

Begin with the spine and neck in good posture, exhale, and fully activate the core.

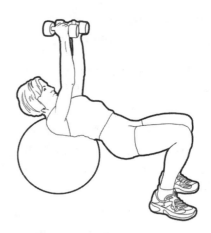

Motion and Stabilization

Slowly begin to inhale; allow the elbows to bend and lower the forearms down while keeping the shoulders from rotating and elbows pointed forward.

Continue to flex the elbows to about 90 degrees, maintaining posture and shoulder and wrist positioning.

Hold; slowly exhale, activate the core, and pull the arms and dumbbells up to the starting point while maintaining posture and elbow and wrist positioning.

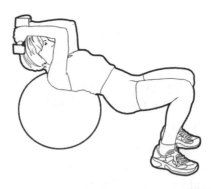

Cable, Overhead Triceps Extension (Lunge Position)

This exercise targets the triceps muscle group. The flexed shoulder position required for this exercise also prelengthens the long-head triceps, keeping them active throughout the range of motion. Performing this exercise in a standing, unbraced position places a high demand for stabilization on the core, trunk, and hip muscles. Although isolated elbow extension and triceps' work might not be considered a functional movement, the stabilization challenges of this exercise are highly transferable to the demands placed on the trunk and hip muscles in certain sport and life activities.

Alignment and Positioning

Hold the straight bar of the upper cable with a shoulder-width grip and step out into a lunge position.

Lean the body forward at the hip as far as needed to stabilize against the pull of the resistance, and externally rotate the shoulders so that the elbow is pointing straight down and locked.

Begin with the spine, shoulders, and neck in good posture and wrists neutral; then exhale and activate the core.

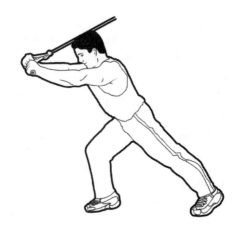

Motion and Stabilization

Slowly begin to inhale; allow the elbows to bend and forearms to be pulled up and back while keeping the shoulders from rotating and elbows pointed down.

Continue to allow the elbows to flex about 90 degrees while maintaining posture and shoulder and wrist positioning.

Hold; slowly exhale, activate the core, and pull the arms and bar to the starting point maintaining posture and elbow and wrist positioning.

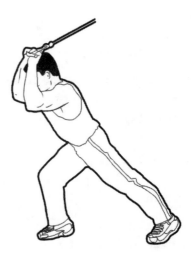

Cable, One-Arm Triceps Extension

This exercise targets the triceps muscle group. The extended shoulder position used for this exercise preshortens the long-head triceps, causing them to become active-insufficient toward the end range of motion. This places more demand on the lateral head of the triceps. Performing this exercise in a standing, nonbraced position will also place some stabilization demand on the core, trunk, and hip muscles. The neutral grip on the handle will also challenge the wrist adductors, which often are a weak link, and help strengthen the wrist overall.

Alignment and Positioning

Face the cable column and grasp the upper cable handle lengthwise with a neutral elbow position and grip.

Lean the body slightly forward at the hips as needed to align the trunk and arms with the cable, and externally rotate the shoulders so that the elbows are pointing back and are fully extended.

Begin with the spine, shoulders, and neck in good posture and wrist neutral; then exhale and fully activate the core.

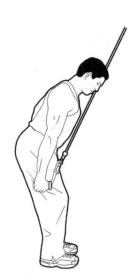

Motion and Stabilization

Slowly begin to inhale; allow the elbows to bend and forearms to be pulled forward and up while keeping the shoulders from rotating and elbows pointed back.

Continue to allow the elbows to flex to about 120 degrees while maintaining posture, shoulder, and wrist positioning.

Hold; slowly exhale, activate the core, and pull the arm and handle to the starting point, maintaining posture and elbow and wrist positioning.

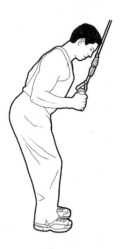

Barbell and Bench, Triceps Press

This exercise targets the triceps and anterior deltoids in a compound pressing movement. The elbow is not designed to work in isolation, making this two-joint exercise a more functional elbow movement. Keeping the arms by the side and working in the median plane limit any significant chest assistance and is a good exercise for developing increased triceps and deltoid strength. However, you should note that the strength increases you obtain while lying on a bench might have little carryover for the pressing movements you perform in sports and life.

Alignment and Positioning

Lay supine on a bench with good posture and the feet braced firmly on the floor or a step.

Pull the shoulder blades slightly together, grasp the bar with a shoulder-width grip, and externally rotate the shoulders so that the elbows are pointing toward the feet and extended.

Begin with good posture, bar over the upper chest, elbows straight, and the core activated.

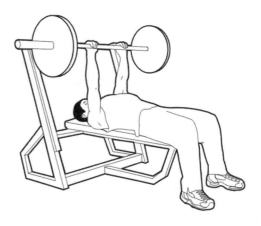

Motion and Stabilization

Slowly begin to inhale; allow the shoulders and elbows to bend and the bar to lower toward the lower sternum, keeping the elbows aligned with the feet.

Continue to lower the bar until the upper arm is almost parallel with the floor, keeping the elbows to the side and maintaining good posture.

Hold; slowly exhale, contract the core, and press the arms and barbell back to the starting position, maintaining proper posture and scapula positioning.

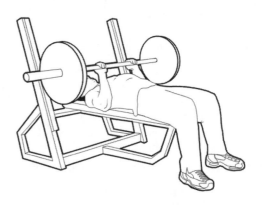

Squat Rack, Triceps Pushup

This exercise also targets the triceps and anterior deltoids in a pressing motion. Performing pushups with a narrower hand position and keeping the arm tight to the side limits chest involvement and forces a similar two-joint movement as the barbell triceps press. The combined shoulder and elbow movement is more functional for loading the elbow extensors; the pushup position also places load on the abdominal and hip flexors for stabilization requirements. You can decrease the challenge by raising or lowering the angle of the body before beginning. Taking one foot from the ground also increases the challenge to the hip flexor and trunk muscles.

Alignment and Positioning

Position the barbell at the desired height for appropriate resistance and place the hands at a shoulder-width grip with the arms extended.

Align the body at a perpendicular angle to the arms with the balls of the feet firmly pressed against the floor.

Begin with good posture; externally rotate the shoulders so that the elbows are pointing toward the feet with the wrists straight and the core activated.

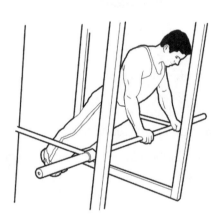

Motion and Stabilization

Slowly begin to inhale; allow the shoulders and elbows to bend lowering the body, keeping the elbows pointed back, and the spine and pelvis stabilized.

Continue to lower the body and move it forward until the lower sternum is over the bar and an approximate 90-degree angle is formed at the elbow.

Hold; slowly exhale, contract the core, and press the body back to the starting position while maintaining proper posture and elbow positioning.

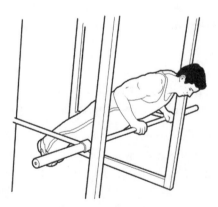

Dumbbell Bicep Flexion

This exercise targets the biceps muscle group. Performing this exercise with dumbbells gives you the choice of working the elbow in a neutral position for more brachioradialis work, or in a supinated position as presented here for more bicep-brachia focus. Isolated elbow flexion and targeted bicep training are not considered functional movements for sport or life demands; however, the high stabilization requirements of the shoulder, scapula, and thoracic spine make this a good exercise for challenging overall posture. I present a technique with this exercise that integrates a slight flexion movement of the shoulder to recruit the anterior deltoids, along with the elbow flexors to reduce elbow stress and assist with postural stabilization.

Alignment and Positioning

Stand with the hips and knees slightly flexed and hold a set of dumbbells next to the body.

Pull the shoulder blades slightly together and position the spine in good posture. Supinate the lower arms so the palms face forward and dumbbells are sideways.

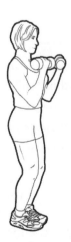

Motion and Stabilization

Begin with the hands and dumbbells just in front of the shoulders, elbows slightly bent, and draw a deep breath.

Slowly begin to exhale; activate the core and flex the shoulders, slightly pulling the arms forward while flexing the elbows; and pulling the lower arms out and up.

Continue to pull the lower arms up just short of the hand being over the elbow, or as far as possible while maintaining posture, shoulder, and wrist positioning.

Hold; then slowly inhale and allow the arms and dumbbells to slowly lower to the starting point while maintaining proper positioning.

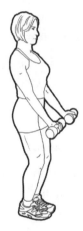

Cable, Overhead Bicep Flexion

This exercise targets the biceps muscle group. Performing this exercise with a flexed shoulder position preshortens the long-head bicep and causes it to become somewhat active-insufficient. This will place more demand on the short-head bicep fibers and will also train shoulder girdle stabilization at a different angle than when working with barbells. Anytime when working the biceps with a straight bar, it is important to grasp the bar with the natural carrying angle in place to avoid additional and potentially detrimental shearing forces across the elbow. This is done by holding the bar at the width naturally created when the shoulders are neutral and the elbows are extended.

Alignment and Positioning

Stand with the hips and knees slightly flexed and grasp the bar of the upper cable with the natural carrying angle in place.

Pull the shoulder blades slightly together and position the spine in good posture.

Align the arms with the upper pulley, begin with the elbows slightly bent, and draw a deep breath.

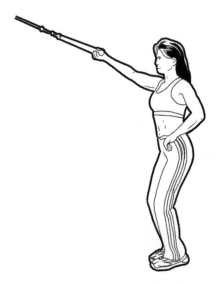

Motion and Stabilization

Slowly begin to exhale; activate the core, flex the shoulders slightly, pulling the arms up, and flex the elbows, pulling the lower arm up and back.

Continue to pull the lower arm up and back as far as possible while keeping posture, shoulder, and wrist positioning.

Hold; slowly inhale and allow the arms and cable to be slowly pulled back to the starting point while maintaining proper positioning.

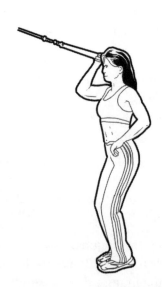

Cable, One-Arm Bicep Flexion (Lunge Position)

This exercise targets the biceps muscle group. Performing this exercise in a standing lunge position places more demand on core, trunk, and hip muscles for stabilization and loads the glutes, associated hip extensors, and quads of the lead leg. You can use different body and shoulder positions to develop different angles of stabilization strength and target different heads of the biceps. For example, by facing away from the cable column and aligning the shoulder in an extended position slightly behind the body, the long-head bicep will stay active throughout the movement, targeting this portion of the biceps. Choose the position and angle appropriate for your goals.

Alignment and Positioning

Grasp the handle of the lower cable and step back into a lunge position, with the trunk leaned at the hip and in good posture.

Pull the shoulder blades slightly together and position the spine in good posture. Supinate the arm so the palm faces forward and wrist is neutral.

Begin with the arm aligned with the cable, elbow slightly bent, and draw a deep breath.

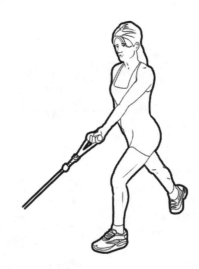

Motion and Stabilization

Slowly begin to exhale; activate the core and flex the shoulder, slightly pulling the arm up while flexing the elbow, and pulling the lower arm out and up.

Continue to pull the lower arm up as far as possible while maintaining posture, and shoulder and wrist positioning.

Hold; slowly inhale and allow the arm and cable to be slowly pulled back to the starting point while maintaining proper positioning.

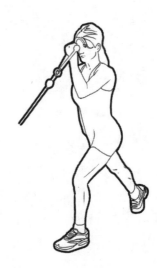

Speed, Agility, and Power Exercises

This chapter presents 34 exercises designed to increase speed, agility, and power. This specific collection of exercises was selected for the best combination of efficiency and safety, as well as for the fact that they can be performed without relying on various special training tools or a partner. These exercises contain specialized movement patterns that will help to develop speed and agility and produce power in all planes of motion. Done properly and consistently as part of a comprehensive training program, these exercises will help to develop the bio-motor abilities most important for optimal performance.

This chapter will begin with exercises designed to develop better hip and knee control for improved foot speed; it will then blend into exercises that require more coordinated movements for greater agility. The exercises then will progress to more plyometric-type movements that teach the body to exploit the stretch reflex for producing optimal power. Finally, several power and med ball exercises will be presented for developing upper torso power in all planes of motion.

The only additional tool presented in this chapter is the medicine ball. Medicine balls come in a variety of sizes and weights and have varying characteristics: Some are made to bounce well; others not at all; and some, such as those I prefer for the following exercises, offer a moderate amount of bounce. Certain manufacturers call the latter balls *power balls;* they provide a sluggish rebound off the ground or a wall, which is ideal for forceful throws when training individually. It is difficult to perform a quick sequence of repetitions with medicine balls that bounce too much or not at all. A medium-size ball is a little smaller than a volleyball, weighing anywhere from about 3 to 5 kilograms, or about 6 to 12 pounds, is recommended for most general power goals.

Here are some training guidelines for performing any of the exercises in this chapter:

1. Always begin with a general warm-up before exercising, such as rope skipping or slow-to-fast progressive sprinting.

2. Perform an entire active stretching or passive active stretching routine following warm-up and preceding exercise.

3. Integrate specific warm-ups and progressive dynamic stretching by performing the first few repetitions of a new exercise more slowly, with less intensity, and smaller range of motion. Gradually increase speed, intensity, and range of movement as you progress through the set.

4. When performing exercises in this chapter, remember that when using an external load (weights or medicine balls), the speed of motion—not the amount of resistance—will promote the development of speed-strength, explosive-strength, and power.

5. Make sure that the integration of these exercises is coordinated with all other forms of training to avoid overtraining and to ensure continued progression toward overall goals.

Speed and Agility Exercises

High Knees

Purpose: This exercise is designed to develop improved stride frequency and quick foot speed. It emphasizes action of the hip flexors and promotes dynamic flexibility of the hip extensors. Improved hip movement and leg power will be helpful for any activity requiring running motions.

Action:

Begin by pulling the knee up as high as possible and exploding off the ground.

Alternate the quick, exaggerated vertical pulling action of each leg.

Pull each leg up as soon as the toe touches the ground and get as many steps in as quickly as possible for a 5- to 10-yard distance.

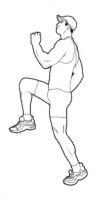 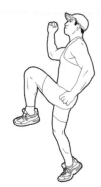 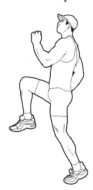

Glute Kickers

Purpose: This exercise improves stride frequency and increased foot speed. It emphasizes action of the knee flexors and promotes dynamic flexibility of the quadriceps.

Action:

Begin with quick leg motion and a pumping action of the arms.

Exaggerate knee flexion and hamstring involvement by attempting to touch the heel to the same-side glute on each stride.

Attempt to pull each leg up as soon as the toe touches the ground and get as many steps in as quickly as possible for a 5- to 10-yard distance.

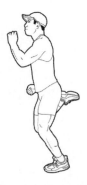 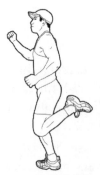 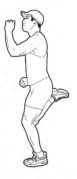

Drum Majors

Purpose: This exercise is designed to help improve stride length. It increases hip flexor strength and improves hip function. It promotes the dynamic flexibility of the hamstrings and hip extensors, and requires additional dynamic stability of the core and trunk muscles to prevent too much posterior pelvic tilting and spinal flexing.

Action:

Begin the running motion with an exaggerated forward kick of the lead leg and lean back slightly.

Pull each leg up as high as possible, keeping it as straight as possible.

Pull each leg up as soon as the toe hits the ground—but try to cover as much distance as possible with each stride—for a 10- to 20-yard distance.

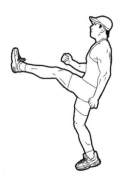
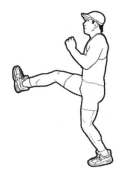
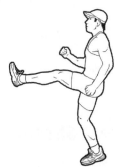

Bounding

Purpose: This exercise is also designed to improve stride length; however, it applies more eccentric loading and exploitation of the stretch reflex for increased power. It promotes additional strengthening and requires more dynamic stability of the ankles and hips. This exercise should probably be integrated following training of vertical jumps and long jumps.

Action:

Begin with a quick running motion, exaggerating the push-off of each stride.

Get as much height and distance with each stride, spending as little time on the ground as possible.

Use exaggerated arm motion to attain greater height and distance.

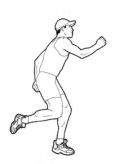
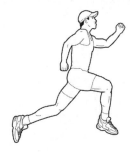
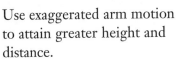
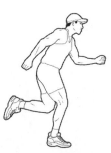

Power Skipping

Purpose: This exercise increases single-leg power for take-offs and single-leg stability for landing. The rhythmic movement is different from running or bounding and requires different coordinated reflex and movement patterns to improve overall agility.

Action:

Perform a single-leg hop off the ground with an explosive movement while reaching up with the same-side arm and opposite leg.

Land on the same side foot to decelerate the body, and then quickly press off the ground with the other foot in an explosive burst, driving the arm up for added lift.

Get as much height on each skip as possible, and use exaggerated arm movements.

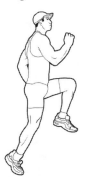 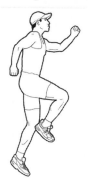 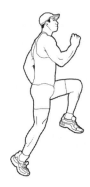

Lateral Shuffle

Purpose: This exercise is designed to develop more efficient lateral movement and dynamic stability of the hips, as well as increase foot speed. The need for quick lateral movement while maintaining a forward orientation of the body with a stable base of support is specific for sports such as tennis or basketball. Certain positions in other sports, such as a linebacker in football or a goalie in soccer, and numerous other competitive or recreational athletes can also benefit from improved lateral movement ability.

Action:

Begin in a ready position with the knees and hips partially flexed and the spine in good posture.

Quickly shuffle to one side with fast stutter steps, keeping the weight on the balls of the feet, shoulders and pelvis squared straight ahead, and eyes forward.

Shuffle for 5 to 10 yards; then plant the outside foot and return while maintaining good posture, shoulder and pelvic positioning, and a lowered center of gravity. Keep a relative shoulder-width stance throughout the movement.

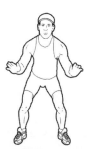 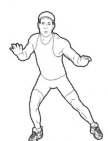 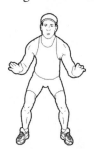

Lateral Crossover Run

Purpose: This exercise teaches a different movement pattern that provides for faster lateral speed. This is necessary to cover longer distances than a shuffle can provide. It also trains for lateral dynamic stability for quick cuts and changes of direction. You can also modify this exercise for diagonal running angles. As with any of these agility exercises, working with a trainer or partner for quick change of direction will improve reaction time and reflex actions of the neuromuscular system.

Action:

Keeping the shoulder square and eyes straight ahead, begin a quick lateral running movement.

The opposite leg to the direction of travel should always cross in front of the other leg. Pump the arms forward and backward in the median plane, allowing the spine and pelvis to turn to promote quicker leg movement that is aligned with the direction of movement.

Run 10 to 20 yards, then plant and quickly come back using the same movement to the opposite side or angle.

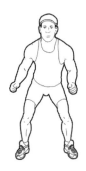 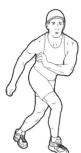 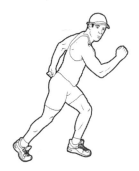

Carioca

Purpose: This exercise is designed to increase agility in the lateral plane. It promotes active flexibility and dynamic stability of the entire pelvic/lumbar/hip complex to provide for the quick pelvic rotations needed for this movement. It might also provide high-speed stepping strategies for improved balance reactions.

Action:

With good posture, the shoulders square, and arms held out to the sides, begin a lateral crossover run technique, pulling the opposite leg to the side of movement in front of the on-side leg.

With the next step, pull the opposite leg behind the on-side leg, focusing on the smooth rotation of the pelvis and lower body, while keeping the shoulders squared and eyes straight ahead.

Alternate the leg movement on each step for about 10 to 20 yards.

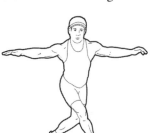 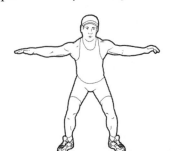 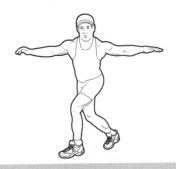

Backpedaling

Purpose: This exercise trains backward movements in the median plane. It emphasizes knee extensor action and challenges the ankle stabilizers for dynamic stability. Most sports and recreational activities require occasional backward movement whether to adjust to a ball or an opponent.

Action:

Begin in good posture and take quick, short steps straight backward while keeping a lowered center of gravity and shoulders squared.

Keep on the balls of the feet and avoid stepping too far back or straightening the body too far up. Backpedal 5 to 10 yards.

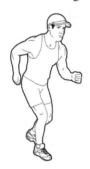 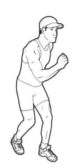 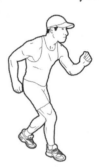

Backpedal Plants with Sprint

Purpose: This exercise further trains backward running; it also challenges metatarsophalangeal (MTP) joint and ankle dynamic stability for the critical planting movement needed to change directions. Most often, backpedaling requires a quick reactive changes of direction to the side or straight forward, as this exercise practices. Be cautious of the intensity of planting and wear proper supportive shoes, as this particular movement is stressful on the MTP joint of the big toe and the plantar fascia.

Action:

Begin with a fast backpedal movement, keeping good posture with the center of gravity lowered and over the toes.

Backpedal for about 5 to 10 yards, or upon a signal, stop abruptly by planting the back foot and pressing the ball of the foot firmly into the ground.

Drive forward in a fast sprinting movement. Sprint forward, plant, and immediately resume a backpedal, making sure to alternate feet for the next plant.

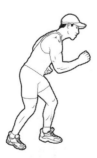 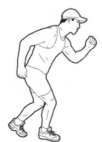 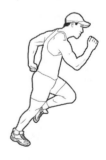

Square Pattern

Purpose: Agility movement patterns combine the various running movements you have learned thus far. You can make multiple combinations other than the ones presented here, depending on need or sport-specific goals. The square pattern integrates lateral movement with forward and backward movements.

Action:
In a 20-yard square, move forward for 5 yards using high knees, glute kicks, sprinting, or other forward movement. Plant and move laterally for 5 yards with a shuffle, crossover, or a carioca movement. Then stop and move backward 5 yards with a backpedal run before planting and moving laterally to the opposite side with a shuffle, crossover, or carioca movement. Repeat or change movement as desired, keeping good form and quick transitions for each movement.

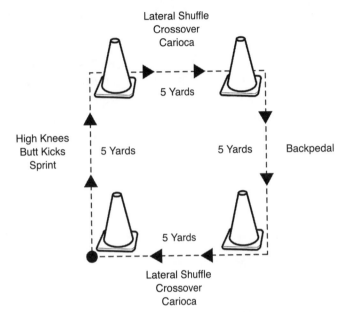

X Pattern

Purpose: This agility pattern combines longer distances at a faster speed to be covered than the square pattern. The X pattern combines both forward diagonal and backward diagonal running with lateral movements. You can change lateral movements as desired for more specificity of motion.

Action:
With a forward orientation of the shoulders and head, begin with a 10-yard diagonal run. Pump the arms forward and backward while allowing the pelvis to rotate toward the direction of motion for faster and more efficient movement. Plant and quickly move laterally for 10 yards with a crossover run, carioca, or shuffle movement. Then plant and begin a fast backward diagonal run while pointing the shoulders and head straight ahead once again. Then plant and move laterally to the original starting point with the desired lateral movement pattern.

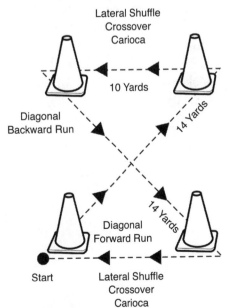

Figure Eight Pattern

Purpose: This agility exercise helps with fast but gradual turning movements. It requires dynamic stability of the ankle, knee, and hip. The smaller and tighter the curve, the more lateral force these areas must be able to stabilize if speed remains constant as compared to larger curves. Begin with short and large (or "fatter") eight patterns, and progress to longer and smaller (or "skinnier") eights.

Action:

Draw or place some cones in a fat figure eight pattern. Run the pattern while increasing intensity on each lap. Be aware of the comparable stability of the outside leg as you round the corners, as well as of the speed reductions you feel you need for stability.

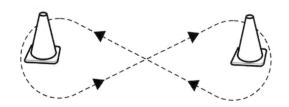

Shuttle Run Patterns

Purpose: The shuttle run can integrate any combinations of forward, backward, lateral, and diagonal running techniques desired. You can also easily plan variable distances for each and further integrate numerous plyometric movements. Try the patterns suggested here, then design others for more goal-specific movements.

Action:

Begin with a 5-yard high knees, then stop and return with a 5-yard backpedal. Start again with a 10-yard power skip followed again by a 10-yard backpedal. Then bound forward for 10 yards, followed quickly by a sprint back for 10 yards.

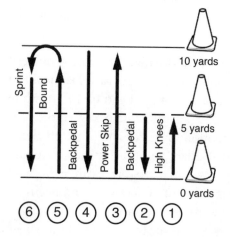

Lower Body Power Exercises

Jump and Reach

Purpose: This is a basic power movement designed to help increase vertical jump height. This exercise integrates maximal hip, trunk, and leg strength into a jumping movement using the stretch reflex. The desired results are primarily increased speed-strength and explosive-strength for increased power and higher jumping ability, which are helpful for numerous sports and activities.

Action:
Begin with a quick drop into a partial squat position, followed by a quick explosive upward jump. Be sure to exaggerate arm movement and allow for an extension of the spine.

Upon landing you may stop to regain balance and begin again, or immediately drop into the next repetition, depending on abilities and goals.

Remember that the goal is typically to achieve maximal heights, not complete maximal repetitions in a certain time.

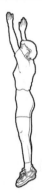

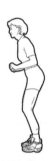

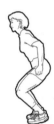

Jump and Tuck

Purpose: This exercise continues power training of the hip and legs musculature but with less assistance of the spinal extensors and shoulder flexors. The tuck at the top requires the use of the arms and flexes the spine, which are opposite actions for assisting with overall height. Adequate height and hang time are necessary to complete this movement.

Action:
Begin with a quick drop into a partial squat position followed by a quick, explosive upward jump. Pull the knees up into the chest and grasp them with the arms.

Hold them for a moment before landing in good posture. Upon landing you may stop to regain balance, then begin again or immediately drop into the next repetition, depending on abilities and goals.

Remember that the goal is again about achieving maximal heights, not maximal repetitions in a certain time.

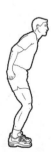

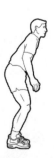

Jump with Glute Kick

Purpose: This exercise continues power training of the hips and legs musculature. However, it requires extra action of the knee flexors, which typically reduces overall vertical jump height. The glute kick at the top requires an adequate height and hang time to complete this movement.

Action:

Begin with a quick drop into a partial squat position followed by a quick explosive upward jump with upward arm action.

As the body ascends, quickly pull the heels to the glutes without accompanying flexion of the hip or forward movement of knees. Hold the heels for a moment before landing in good posture.

Upon landing you may momentarily stop and begin again, or immediately drop into the next repetition.

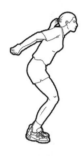
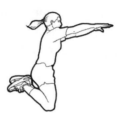
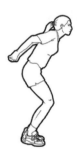

Twist Jump

Purpose: This exercise integrates the vertical jump with controlled spinal rotation. The twisting motion performed in mid-air allows for a low-resisted rotational movement that recruits the trunk, oblique, and spinal muscles responsible for accelerating and decelerating spinal rotation. This will help to prepare the body for more forceful rotational actions used in a variety of sports. It also develops dynamic-flexibility, dynamic-stability, and impact-stability of the trunk and pelvis for the repeated landings in a rotated position.

Action:

Begin from a symmetrical stance with good posture and perform a quick vertical hop followed by a controlled twisting movement of the pelvis and lower body.

Land with the shoulders square, facing forward and the feet parallel pointing about 30 degrees to the side. Upon landing, immediately hop again while performing a controlled rotation back to neutral, or land completely to a 30-degree position to the opposite side.

Repeat for the desired reps. Keep vertical height low to reduce impact forces and focus more on the rotational movement.

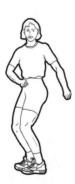
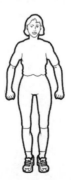
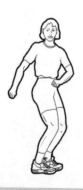

Lunge Jump

Purpose: This exercise trains power of the hips, trunk, and legs musculature from an asymmetrical position. The positioning different from the basic vertical jump requires different synergetic actions of the legs for both the explosive concentric movement and for the eccentric dynamic stabilization of the landing. The additional challenge and perpendicular momentum of the legs will reduce overall vertical jump height, making arm action highly important for completion of this movement.

Action:

Begin with a quick drop into a lunge position and a cocking action of the arms, followed by a quick, explosive upward jump throwing the arms up and reaching toward the sky.

As the body ascends, quickly pull the back leg forward and forward leg back in a scissor movement so as to land back in a lunge position to the opposite side.

Upon landing you may momentarily stop and begin again, or immediately drop into the next repetition depending on your ability and goals.

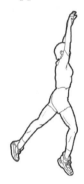
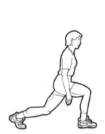
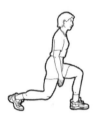

Long Jumps (Hops)

Purpose: This exercise trains the hips, trunk, and legs musculature for a more forward power and movement as opposed to vertical. However, for maximal distance, you still need adequate height. This exercise should probably precede the bounding movement presented in an earlier section, because a bound is more or less a one-leg hop for distance. Because distance is the goal for this movement, arm action is again important for maximal performance.

Action:

Begin with a quick drop into a partial squat position and a cocking action of the arms.

Immediately perform a quick explosive forward and upward jump, throwing the arms up and out. As the body travels up and forward, quickly pull the legs forward and reach out with them, landing on the heels.

Upon landing you may momentarily stop and begin again, or immediately continue in long hopping motions, depending on your ability and goals.

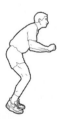
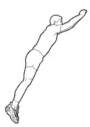
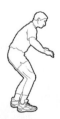

Triple Jumps

Purpose: This exercise requires a much higher level of coordination and control than the long jumps. There is an increased requirement for speed-strength, explosive-strength, and dynamic-stability, as each leg will be loaded isolaterally. You should train vertical jumping and long jumping with single-leg take-offs and landings before integration of this exercise. You can also add a preceding running movement to load the first jump, which increases overall distance.

Action:

Begin in a standing position (or progress to a running start) and perform a quick long jump landing on one foot. Immediately press off with that foot, jumping out as far as possible, and land on the other foot. Again press off with that foot to make the final jump out as far as possible, and finish with a two-point landing. The sequence is a two-leg jump, a one-leg jump, and an alternate leg jump with a two-feet landing. You may stop and go again from a standing position or begin the run for the next repetition. You can also simply continue without stopping, because the ending is the same position as the start.

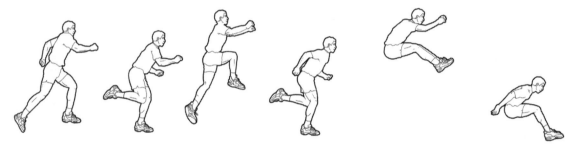

Lateral Jumps

Purpose: This exercise trains power of the hip, trunk, and legs musculature for a lateral movement. It can be performed with a distance emphasis or a height emphasis. Cones can be used to set goal distance; hurdles, benches, or other objects could be used for achieving height goals. This exercise requires more lateral stability of the ankles and knees, particularly when greater distances are attempted as opposed to height.

Action:

Begin with a quick drop into a partial squat position and a cocking action of the arms.

Immediately perform a quick explosive lateral and upward jump, throwing the arms up and over. As the body travels up and sideways, quickly pull the legs up and extend them out to the other side for landing.

Upon landing, you may momentarily stop and begin again or immediately continue in lateral hopping motions, depending on your ability and goals.

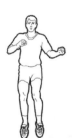

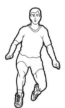

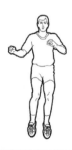

Single-Leg Lateral Jumps

Purpose: This exercise requires more lateral explosive strength and power, as well as increased levels of dynamic stability of the ankles and knees. More stability requirements accompany greater lateral movement, as opposed to vertical. Therefore, you should perform the exercise with the proper combination of each. Cones can be used to set distance goals while hurdles, benches, or other objects could be used for achieving height goals.

Action:

Begin with a quick drop into a partial squat position and a cocking action of the arms. Immediately press off with the outside foot for a quick lateral and upward jump, throwing the arms up and over.

As the body travels up and over, quickly position the other leg for the landing and quick lateral bound back to the starting leg.

This lateral bounding movement can be performed in a strict lateral plane or combined with forward movement, depending on goal specificity.

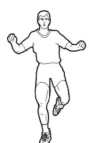
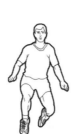
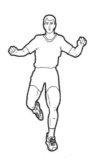

Hexagon Jump Pattern

Purpose: This exercise integrates multiple combinations of the jumping exercises previously presented, as well as of the variations not presented. Combining different jumps pushes the neuromuscular system for integration of previously stored motor patterns, muscle synergies for productions of power, and multiple stabilization strategies.

Action:

Draw or mark a hexagon shape with each side being about two feet. Begin with a forward vertical jump to the center of the hexagon. Upon landing, immediately rebound at a diagonal angle, only to rebound again to the center of the hexagon. Proceed to a lateral jump and continue around the octagon until all 12 jumps have been completed. You can also perform this exercise with a single-leg hop version.

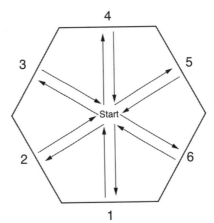

Upper Body Power Exercises

Med Ball, Forward Pass

Purpose: This exercise begins the integration of the arms for explosive power. It does not incorporate as much trunk and lower body actions as subsequent exercises, but does provide the basic push pattern used in several sports and activities. It also allows you to get familiar with the characteristics of the ball.

Action:

Begin in a shallow squat position, with the hands holding on to the sides of the ball and close to the chest in preparation for a forward passing motion.

Quickly press out of the squat position in a jumping-like motion, rising to the balls of the feet while forcefully pushing the ball out and up, releasing the ball approximately at a 90-degree angle.

Catch the ball after it bounces once off the ground following its rebound off the wall, and repeat the movement.

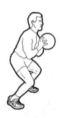
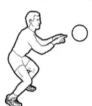
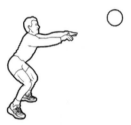

Med Ball, Forward Underhand Throw

Purpose: Throwing with maximal power requires the coordinated actions of the entire body. Try to use the arms as extensions of the spine that simply transfer the body's force and direct the release of the projectile. This exercise further links shoulder movement with the entire extensor chain of the trunk and lower body, much like the jump and reach. However, it is the force of the throw that's the focus, not the height of the jump.

Action:

Begin with a quick drop into a partial squat position, pulling the arms down between the legs and holding the ball with an underhand grasp.

Immediately press out of the squat position in a jumping motion, forcefully pulling the arms forward and up and releasing the ball at an approximate 45-degree angle.

Catch the ball after it bounces once off the ground and after its rebound off the wall, and repeat the movement.

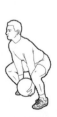
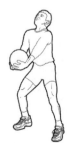
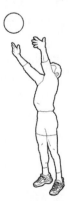

Med Ball, Forward Overhand Throw

Purpose: This exercise links an overhead throwing movement with the power of the trunk and hip flexors. This general throwing movement increases speed strength of the latissimus dorsi and associated shoulder extensors. It also increases power of the trunk and hip flexors and eccentric deceleration abilities of the spinal erector system. Overhand throwing is more transferable than underhand variations for most sporting activities. One arm throwing with smaller med balls may be even better for sports specificity.

Action:

Begin in a ready position and step forward while extending the spine and pulling the ball back over the head.

Leading with the chest, perform a whipping movement by quickly flexing the spine and forcefully pulling the arms overhead, releasing the ball slightly higher than a 90-degree angle.

Catch the ball directly after its rebound off the wall or after it bounces once off the ground, then repeat.

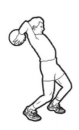 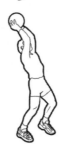 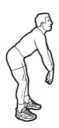

Med Ball, Forward Pullover Throw

Purpose: This exercise is designed to continue developing speed strength and explosive-strength of the trunk and hip flexors. It also uses more lats for initiation and follow-through of the movement. The rectus abdominus is primarily a fast-twitch muscle designed to initiate powerful movements of the extremities. However, ballistic spinal flexion, particularly when performed in a seated position, is stressful to lumbar disks; it is not recommended for everyone to perform this exercise. Also, remember that high-intensity, fast-twitch muscle training should be low in volume, so keep repetitions low and sets moderate on this exercise.

Action:

Lay in a supine position with the ball grasped for an overhead throwing motion.

Lead with a quick overhead pulling motion of the arms, followed by a quick activation of the trunk and hip flexors in a situp motion.

Release the ball approximately at a 65- to 70-degree angle and hold this position. Catch the ball directly after its rebound off the wall or after it bounces once off the ground, then repeat.

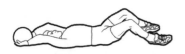 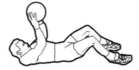

Med Ball, Backward Underhand Throw

Purpose: This exercise provides for probably the most powerful throwing movement possible by harnessing the full power of the entire trunk and lower body extensor chain. This general underhand throwing movement occurs in a modified pattern for several strength competitions, such as the famous Camber Throw of the Scotland games. However, this exercise has a backward release and a jumping movement to get maximal force behind the throw.

Action:

Begin with a quick drop into a partial squat position while pulling the arms down between the legs and holding the ball with an underhand grasp.

Immediately explode out of the squat position in a jumping motion. Simultaneously, forcefully pull the arms up and over the head, releasing the ball approximately at a 45-degree angle, depending on the height of the rebound wall.

Turn quickly and catch the ball as it rebounds off the wall or on the first bounce off the ground following the rebound.

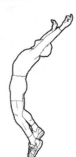

Med Ball, Lateral Throw

Purpose: This exercise begins the integration of ballistic rotational movements of the trunk and entire body. Although these movements can be stressful to vertebral disks and the surrounding tissues, as well as the knees, they are a part of all sports and life. Rotational power is at the heart of performance for numerous sports such as baseball, football, golf, hockey, tennis, and boxing—just to name a few. They are also found in life movements such as chopping wood, bucking hay bails, or throwing a rock. Proper form and progression of rotational movements are vital.

Action:

Begin in a shallow squat position with good posture and twist the body to cock it to one side while holding the ball in a slightly underhand grasp.

Quickly unrotate the trunk and pull the ball around the body, keeping the arms straight but loose and not locked. Allow the opposite side hip to rotate slightly in with the rotation of the body and the foot to internally pivot on the ball of the foot.

Release the ball at a 90-degree angle and hold this position to catch the ball on its first bounce off the ground following the rebound from the wall.

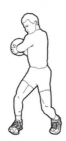
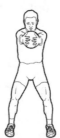
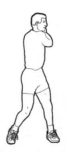

Hang Clean

Purpose: The hang clean can be used to create high levels of power in even a faster amount of time, with less assisted jumping movement as used for most med-ball exercises. This movement is designed for starting strength and speed strength, making the speed of movement of fundamental importance and the weight load of less importance. Remember that this movement is a lower body exercise with trunk and upper body assistance, and could have been easily placed in the lower body section.

Action:

Begin with good posture in a shallow squat position. Hold the bar against the upper thighs with an overhand, shoulder-width grasp.

Quickly drop a few inches and explode back up, extending the knees and hips while quickly pulling the bar up, keeping it close to the body. Allow the body and bar to continue to rise until the toes are almost off the ground, and then quickly drop back into a partial squat position while flipping the elbows underneath the bar.

Catch the bar on the upper chest with the elbows pointing out. Stand the rest of the way up, then lower the bar back in a controlled reverse movement and repeat.

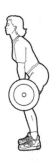 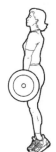 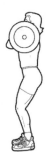

Power Clean

Purpose: The power clean has long been a primary exercise for most sport-training programs and has general movement pattern carryover. However, unless you are training for Olympic-type competitions, there is no direct transference to any sport, so focus on technique, not weight load and integrate this exercise only after mastering squats, dead-lifts, med ball backward underhand throws, and hang cleans.

Action:

Begin in a deep, narrow squat position with the spine in as close to a natural arch as possible. If the spine is too rounded, try beginning with the plates resting on blocks or select a different exercise. Hold the bar with the arms outside the legs with an overhand, shoulder-width grasp. Quickly drive up from the squat position, while quickly pulling the bar up, keeping it close to the body. Allow the body and bar to continue rising until the toes are almost off the ground, and then quickly drop back into a partial squat position while flipping the elbows underneath to catch the bar. Stand the rest of the way up, then lower the bar back in a controlled reverse movement and repeat.

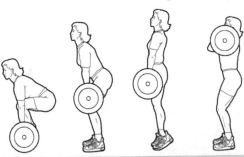

Push-Press (Jerk)

Purpose: This is a power exercise designed for overhead explosive strength and pressing power. It integrates vital lower body power, which is the key to the movement. Therefore, do not think of this as a simple military press for strengthening the shoulders. Technique and speed are more important than weight load.

Action:

Stand in good posture with the bar resting on the upper chest and elbows pointing straight ahead.

Quickly drop into a shallow squat position and immediately explode back up while pressing the bar up.

Continue to drive the body and bar up until the toes are almost off the ground; then drop back down while locking out the elbows. Hold; then bring the bar back down to the original starting position in a controlled movement.

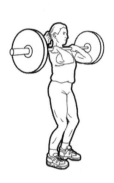 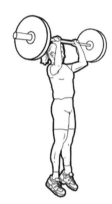 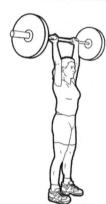

Power Pushup

Purpose: This exercise promotes explosive strength and speed strength development of the pushing muscles of the upper body. It also requires dynamic stability of the shoulder, scapula, and wrist.

Action:

Begin in a normal pushup position with the hands set just outside shoulder width. Drop quickly to a point where the arms form approximately a 90-degree angle and the upper arm is almost parallel to the floor.

Immediately explode back up with enough force for the extended arms to be well off the ground. Try to land with the hands in the same original starting position, then repeat.

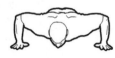 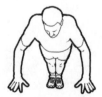 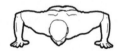

Progressive Program Design

Some people may be able to achieve reasonable progression toward their goals and avoid short-term training injuries simply through a random selection of exercises for each muscle group—as long as their exercise technique is adequate. Chapter 4, "Resistance Training Technique," discussed the important role exercise technique plays in reaching your overall goals. However, without proper program design, ultimate goals and optimal performance are most likely unobtainable, and increased structural wear on the body is likely despite good technique. Muscular imbalances, strain of connective tissues, and mechanical wear patterns often result from repeated performance of inefficiently designed programs.

A training program should seek to improve all bio-motor abilities in proportion to the needs and overall goals of the individual through the systematic manipulation of acute program variables.[2, 7, 21] The program should strive to improve function and overall health, yet still allow for the pursuit of performance or cosmetic goals. You should sacrifice neither function nor long-term health needs when training for short-term sporting goals or to achieve dramatic changes in physical appearance. Too often people will compromise balanced fitness to obtain these types of temporary rewards. As a former professional athlete, competitive power lifter, and bodybuilder, I am very aware of how overall fitness can be sacrificed for personal athletic and cosmetic desires.

A person's needs should be the first focus of an integrated fitness and performance program. Needs are best determined through an in-depth assessment from a skilled practitioner. You can reach goals only at the level supported by the fitness base. The bio-motor capabilities that comprise the base are strength, endurance, stability, and mobility. Once the body has been strengthened and stabilized and has attained adequate balance, flexibility, and endurance, you can safely and efficiently pursue training for other abilities more directly related to athletic performance.

This chapter provides a system for developing progressive exercise programs intended to improve the body within the proper hierarchy of addressing needs prior to accomplishing goals. The following figure depicts the relationship of the seven bio-motor abilities. It is presented here again to reemphasize the importance of this training concept before delving into the exercise programming. This hierarchal training philosophy is at the core of all the programs presented in this chapter.

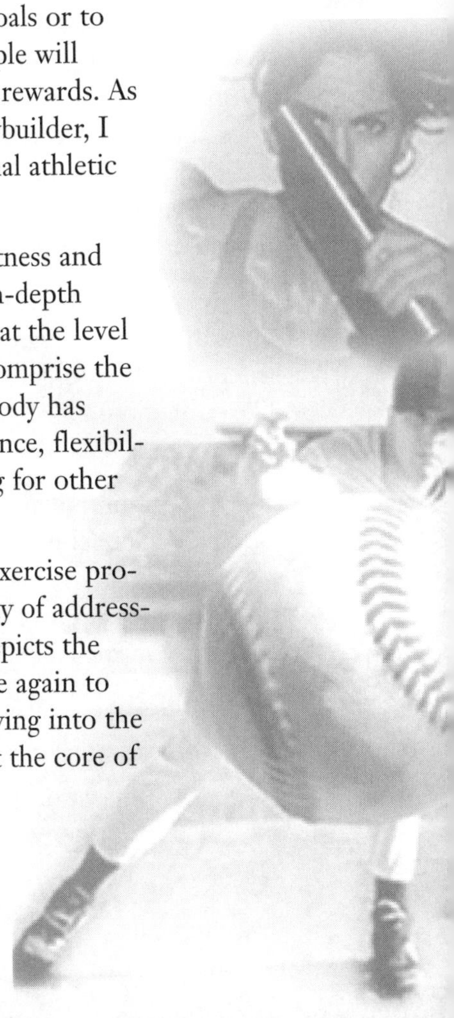

An exercise program, most simply stated, is a collection of exercises grouped together into routines and performed with a certain amount of volume for a specific amount of time. However, you can assemble an endless combination of exercises and techniques for any program. You can also perform these exercises with an infinite number of intensities, repetitions, sets, and tempos, sequenced in any manner imaginable. With so many programming options available, it is important to establish systems to adjust all these numerous program variables. I will begin by defining the major variables for exercise programming.

Program Design Variables

The science of program design requires the use of established knowledge of the designed structure and functions of the human body,

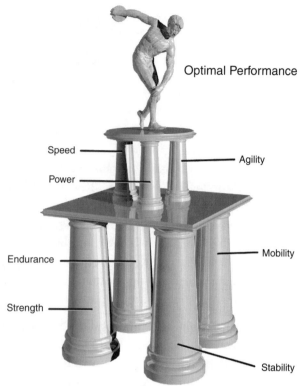

The seven bio-motor abilities for optimal performance.

as well as its adaptations to different exercise stimuli. Although it would take volumes of books to present all the physiological and biomechanical information pertaining to human performance and adaptation, the basic facts presented in Chapter 1, "The Human Body: Anatomical Design and Function," provide enough information to understand the programming criteria used here. By presenting a few sound principles, I can offer a concise summary of the most pertinent information for designing exercise programs and adjusting acute variables.

True principles always have a scientific foundation, have been field tested, can be reproduced, and are recognized by the majority of the experts in the related field of study. Some of the principles presented herein for manipulating program variables come in part from the likes of famous strength coach Charles Poliquin and well-known researchers of strength and conditioning William Kraemer and Steven Fleck.

You can find identical and similar principles of program design in the resources of Baechle, Bompa, Chek, Chu, Clark, Foran, and Gambetta. Some of the commonalities these experts present address the need to systematically manipulate certain program variables to experience optimal results. These primary variables determine the effectiveness of any program. I will discuss them in their interdependent relationships and present them in the following order:

1. Intensity
2. Volume, consisting of:
   * Repetitions   * Duration   * Tempo
   * Sets   * Frequency
3. Recovery
4. Sequence

Intensity

Intensity is probably the most important program variable to consider when designing an exercise program. It is defined as the level of effort exerted as compared to the maximal effort possible. In resistance training, this is the measurement of the load as compared to what could be successfully lifted in one maximal effort. It is often expressed as a percentage of one repetition maximum, or %1RM.

Therefore, if a person performs repetitions of an exercise with 70 percent of what he could maximally lift with a single attempt, we would classify this as 70%1RM. Remember that maximal strength and efforts do not need to be attempted to determine a percentage of 1RM. Close estimates can be made from completion of submaximal sets. For example, what you can perform with maximal effort for 6 reps equals approximately 85% of 1RM.[8] This will vary somewhat depending on the exercise movement, the muscle type being tested, and the individual; but overall, this is a fairly accurate estimate.

The level of intensity required to bring about any training effect has to do with the *principle of progressive overload*, which states that you must supply sufficient intensity and duration to overload the muscle's present levels of adaptation to improve strength or endurance.[21, 22] The key word here is "sufficient," which does not mean having to train to absolute failure to make gains. Often it takes several cycles to estimate what is "sufficient" in the context of individual adaptive abilities; this changes as the athlete progresses. For this reason, you should perform a continual assessment process at the end of each program to determine the effectiveness of the efforts and intensity levels that were utilized.

The intensity level or amount of load that you have chosen will affect all other training variables. The intensity or load can also influence all elements of technique and might require optional changes in positioning, stabilization choices, and tempo. The amount of intensity will also ultimately determine the energy systems that you use and the muscle fiber types that will be recruited.

It is also important to note that as intensity or the external load increases, so does the requirement to generate greater internal force, which proportionally increases the amount of stress to all soft-tissue and joint surfaces, regardless of whether this is desired. Therefore, any change in intensity should be an intentional action, a preplanned part of the training system that is consistent with all other variables and training goals. The athlete should understand its relationship to other variables to make the proper adjustments as intensity changes for each training phase or cycle.

Intensity's relationship to volume probably is the most critical to understand, as there are so many components of volume. Overall, most authors agree that there are strong reasons to decrease total volume as intensity increases.[16, 27, 41] The major disagreement among the experts is in how much volume should be decreased, and in what manner it should be done. One component of volume that needs no thought for adjustment is the amount of repetitions performed. As intensity increases, repetitions automatically decrease, leading to the desired end of decreased total volume. However, the other components of volume are not as easy to manipulate because they all require voluntary choices.

The number of sets performed is a complete choice and one that is often overlooked. As intensity increases and repetitions decrease, the number of sets should increase. This is particularly true when any increase in muscle mass is desired. Maintaining or decreasing sets along with decreased repetitions would lead to an overreduction of total volume. Steep drops in volume not only cause a lack of sufficient stimulation for muscle hypertrophy, they don't provide enough work for motor unit fatigue, which is important for hypertrophy and highly essential for improvements in strength for more advanced individuals.[16, 27, 28]

Also, workouts too low in total volume will not elicit the type of hormonal responses that are conducive to gains in hypertrophy, or increased exercise post-oxygen consumption (EPOC), which temporarily raises metabolic activity.[8, 21] In other words, low-volume workouts won't build as much muscle or burn as many calories during, and more important, for the several hours following, the workout. This typically defeats the purposes usually involved with the original decision for increasing intensity in the first place.

Tempo is another component of volume, because it directly affects the total amount of time under tension. Therefore, you should also consider changes in tempo when raising intensity. When you use heavier loads, there is inherently more inertia involved, which becomes increasingly difficult to overcome, particularly when you increase momentum. Simply stated, it is more difficult to control heavier loads when they are moved faster. Often, a reduction in the speed of movement accompanies increased loads to maintain critical elements of exercise technique, such as stability, positioning, and optimal range of motion. This is precisely why tempo is one of the elements of exercise technique, as well as being an important variable of program design.

The total amount of exercises selected for any body part also affects total volume for those muscles involved. When increasing intensity, decreasing reps, adding sets, and using slower tempos, it is also logical to reduce the number of exercises per body part. This not only maintains proper ratios of volume and intensity, it also allows for the extra recovery needed when working with heavier loads.

As intensity increases, so does the demand on the neural system. It is well documented that the recovery of nerve cells takes at least five to six times as the recovery of muscle cells.[27] In certain high-intensity strength training phases, it is not uncommon to rest for five to eight minutes between sets. This allows for close-to-complete neural, as well as metabolic, recovery.

Often, active recovery is an alternative to complete rest; you can accomplish this by performing supersets with movement patterns that are opposite from, or unrelated to, the previous movement. This still allows for adequate recovery of the specific motor units previously recruited and supplies more opportunity for increased overall work. This is a logical choice in certain phases because usually there are other exercises and training goals that must be accomplished during the session.

The following table demonstrates the specific adjustments to the various components of volume and changes in recovery as intensity is increased.

Volume and Recovery Adjustments for Increased Intensity

Training Goals	Intensity	Repetitions	Sets	Sub Total #1	Tempo Assignment	Sub Total #2	# Exercises/ Muscle Grp	Initial Volume	Rest Between Sets
Endurance	X	17	2	34 reps	2111 (5 secs)	170 secs	3	520 secs	30–60 secs
Hypertrophy	X + Y	10	3	30 reps	3121 (7 secs)	210 secs	2	420 secs	60–240 secs
Strength	X + Y + Z	5	5	25 reps	4122 (9 secs)	225 secs	1	225 secs	300+ secs

Intensity can also affect the duration and frequencies of a workout, which are additional components of total volume. Keep higher-intensity workouts under one hour, and possibly even less. This recommendation is based on several studies that have shown that increases in testosterone and growth hormone levels peak after about 40 minutes of intense exercise.[21] You may wish to spend any spare time following the workout on active stretching or low-intensity endurance and cardiovascular training. Massage and myofascia release can also be a good follow-up to a high-intensity workout.

It may also be beneficial to reduce the frequency of workouts during high-intensity training phases. Heavy loads are more likely to stress connective tissue, which takes two to three times longer to recover than muscle tissue.[16, 28, 41] However, many people do not have the flexibility in their training schedule to adjust frequency without missing sessions all together. In these cases, design routines that allow muscles targeted in prior sessions to be de-emphasized in subsequent sessions during high-intensity phases.

The intensity level of an exercise will also dictate its preferred placement in the sequence of the routine. The higher the intensity level, the more the neural demand, and the earlier in the routine it would be logically placed. However, certain biomechanical factors, such as the exercise's effect on stabilizers needed for following movements, or the priority of overall goals, occasionally cause a change to this sequencing guideline.

It is also quite reasonable to purposely spread intense exercises throughout the routine rather than place them all at the beginning. This would require a more consistent level of effort throughout the routine and feasibly promote a more consistent hormonal response. This is preferable for most people when compared to routines that quickly elevate lactic acid and hormonal response, and then allow them to plummet as the workout wanes. In any case, keep in mind that the further along high-intensity exercises are placed in the sequence of a routine, the more difficult they become.

Volume

Volume for a muscle is the total amount of time it is under tension. It can be broken down into *initial volume* (total amount of time under tension for a given muscle during a single routine) and total volume. You can calculate initial volume by multiplying the number of repetitions by the set and then by the tempo of each rep. You would need to consider each movement that targets that area to determine initial volume.

Total volume can be further described in weekly, monthly, or yearly periods. You can calculate it for a given phase, mesocycle, or macrocycle simply by multiplying the initial volume of a routine by the frequency it was performed during the phase or cycle desired. Tracking volume is a simple matter of disciplined record keeping, which is much easier when the program preplans and directs the proper amounts of desired volume for each muscle group for each routine. This preplanning and calculation ensure that proper volumes are obtained simply by following the workouts already drawn up.

Probably the most critical component of volume is the number of repetitions performed. This is the first variable you should consider when designing an exercise program. Although I have cited intensity as the most important program variable, it is the prior selection of the desired repetitions and the total duration of the set that should determine the amount of intensity you should use. In other words, use the preplanned number of repetitions to select the necessary weight loads, as opposed to selecting desired weight loads and simply letting the repetitions adjust themselves.[27, 28]

The number and tempo of the repetitions determine the duration of a set; therefore, they dictate the energy systems and muscle fiber types that will be trained. This will also determine the types of adaptations the neuromuscular system will experience. A continuum of neural-to-metabolic changes takes place within the neuromuscular system based on the level of intensity and the duration of the given set. More neural, intramuscular adaptations occur with sets performed with low repetitions and high intensities. Conversely, more cellular, metabolic adaptations of the muscle result from prolonged sets or greater amounts of time under tension.

Sets that are designed for performance of only a few repetitions would obviously necessitate the use of higher intensities and would require more use from the short-term energy system, or ATP-CP. This would also stimulate recruitment of more type IIB muscle fibers, which would be more appropriate for strength and power goals. Sets performed in the mid-ranges of repetitions would require more contributions from the glycolitic or lactic acid energy systems. This would target the various types of IIA fibers, which are designed for a blend of strength and endurance and are associated with the greatest increases in hypertrophy of the muscle.

Sets that are designed to be performed in high repetition ranges would work better for the aerobic or oxidative energy system and require more activation of type IIC and type I muscle fibers. This energy system and these muscle fibers are ideal for use in activities requiring greater levels of muscular endurance. The following table depicts the relationships of time under tension with the corresponding energy systems and muscle fiber types. It also shows the neural-metabolic continuum of adaptation to time under tension and the relative training goals that would be appropriate at each point.

The Neural-Metabolic Continuum of Adaptation to Time Under Tension

Energy System (Continuum)	Primary Muscle Fiber Types Stimulated	Time under Tension	Neural-Metabolic Adaptation (Continuum)	Specific Training Goals	Suggested Recovery Between Sets
ATP-PC	IIB	1–10 secs (1–2 reps)*	Neural Adaptation	Strength/Power	5+ min
↓	IIaB	↓		Strength-Hypertrophy	↓
Glycolitic/ Lactic Acid	IIAB IIAb IIA	30–90 secs (6–15 reps)*		Hypertrophy	1–4 min
↓	IIAC IIC	↓	↓	Hypertrophy-Endurance	↓
Oxidative/ Aerobic	IC I	180 + secs (30+ reps)*	Metabolic Adaptations	Endurance	0–30 secs

*Average tempo of 6 seconds

By using this table, you can accomplish the proper duration of any set for the desired training goals by simply selecting the amount of resistance required to be challenged during the listed time under tension. Estimates of the number of repetitions performed that correspond to the targeted amount of time under tension are also given. However, these numbers assume that an average tempo of six seconds per repetition is utilized. More or less reps can be produced in the same amount of time under tension, with no change in adaptations, simply by adjusting the tempo.

For example, a set of 5 repetitions performed with a 10-second tempo should provide nearly identical physiological adaptations as performing 10 repetitions with a 5-second tempo. Therefore, independent changes in repetitions or tempos will not significantly affect physiological adaptations as long as the total duration of a set remains the same.

We have assumed that the amount of time under tension was performed with intensity levels that were close to causing momentary muscular failure. However, at certain times it might be desirable to perform low repetitions with lighter loads. Ballistic movements such as plyometric and medicine ball–throwing exercises do not need maximal loads to accomplish their purpose.

Exercises of high complexity that require greater amounts of neural drive and specific intermuscular coordination, such as a power clean or the snatch, are often trained with reduced loads for technique development of the movement itself, unless training for competitive use of the exercise. It is best to perform fewer repetitions with lighter loads and avoid any muscular failure when first learning new movement patterns that demand high levels of cognitive control. Proper motor pattern development may be impended with higher repetitions or heavier loads, as small, often unnoticeable compensations can begin as certain stabilizers and synergists fatigue.[27]

The tempo of a repetition has a much more dramatic training effect than simply its contribution to volume. Tempo is also a part of technique and can have a definitive influence on the specific type of strength that will be developed. Intrafusal muscle fibers, or muscle spindles, are sensitive to the speed of muscle contraction. They relay detailed information pertaining to changes in the length and tension of the muscles to the appropriate level of the control system for processing. Once information on speed of contraction, speed of force productions, and rates of acceleration is learned and stored in the control system, specific intramuscular adaptations can be recalled and used for similar demands in appropriate situations.

Basically, this means that there are tempos more suited for achieving specific strength gains such as maximal strength, static strength, explosive strength, and speed strength, including both of starting strength and acceleration strength. Chapter 4, "Resistance Training Technique," gave a more detailed account of how tempo is altered as an element of exercise technique to achieve the different types of specific training adaptations.

The science of volume prescription continues when selecting the appropriate number of sets per exercise or per body part. Sets are always a total option, regardless of intensity levels or repetitions. Contemporary literature provides recommendations ranging from 1 to 12 sets, depending on the goals. With such an abundance of options available, it is important to look at physiological factors for basing decisions for prescribing sets.

As previously discussed, there should typically be an inverse relationship between the sets and number of repetitions performed, and a correlating relationship of sets with changes in intensity. Adding sets to maintain adequate levels of volume as intensity increases is critical if you want positive hormonal responses, increased EPOC, and gains in strength or hypertrophy. This principle of increasing sets proportionally with increases in intensity is occasionally altered for special cases when increased strength is needed along with a maintenance or decrease in muscle size.

For example, consider a competitive wrestler needing to stay under a certain weight class. Think of a female dancer or gymnast who could use additional strength and power, but cannot afford to have larger glutes and thighs. In these situations, high-intensity and any hypertrophy phases are coupled with greater reductions in volume by adjusting the amount of sets. This way it is still possible to develop strength and power while avoiding unwanted hypertrophy.

Muscle size and gender should also affect the number of sets selected. Larger muscles typically respond better to more sets than smaller muscles. Larger people tend to benefit from more sets than smaller people.[27] The average male responds better to more sets than the average female.[16] It is also logical to consider muscle composition for prescribing sets. Muscles composed of primarily fast-twitch fibers are developed better with more sets, as slow-twitch muscles are stimulated best with less sets.[8, 16, 27]

This information supports the intensity-rep-set relationships already proposed, as fast-twitch muscles also respond better to higher intensity levels with fewer repetitions, whereas the slow-twitch muscles are better worked with lighter loads and high repetitions. The programs presented later in this chapter provide examples of how these recommendations on selecting the number of sets are integrated throughout the different cycles and phases of training.

Research and practical experience have shown that beginners often benefit in strength from one or two sets no matter the gender of the person or the size and fiber types of the muscles. Nor does it seem to make dramatic differences whether the sets are low- or high-rep. The key here is more about the quality of the sets rather than the quantity. This is attributed to the initial neural adaptations to the new motor patterns and the inter- and intramuscular changes that quickly occur. This is the reason studies on exercise programming—or on fitness devices—that use primarily sedentary people as the test subjects are inconclusive and unreliable. This effect soon levels out as a person progresses and adapts to the present training loads and volumes. It is then that proper systematic planning of sets and coordination of reps, intensity, and recovery all become more critical for achieving significant results.

Duration and frequency are other components of volume you should plan for when designing exercise programs. *Duration* is a general term that describes almost any portion of volume. For example, you can obviously calculate the duration of a set by multiplying the amount of reps by the average tempo. You could also simply incorporate a stopwatch, as many trainers do, to record the actual duration of the set.

Recommended duration of sets is again based on the neural-metabolic continuum and the associated training goals. Duration could also pertain to the time period of a given routine, as discussed previously when I recommended an hour or even less per training session to maintain a positive hormonal response. However, this might need to be adjusted according to the person's conditioning, abilities, needs, overall goals, or the presence of an uncontrolled variable such as illness, mental stress, or diet. Duration might be associated with the length of a training cycle or phase and can be expressed in days, weeks, months, or even years. Recommendations on these will be presented later in this chapter in the "Periodization and Progression" section.

Frequency, like duration, is a general term that for our purposes relates to how often an exercise, routine, phase, or cycle is performed. The frequency of any exercise is dependent on several factors such as the newness of the exercise, its complexity, or its deemed importance for addressing needs or accomplishing goals. You must perform an exercise often enough—particularly if it is new or highly complex—to develop and store the specifics of the motor program. Too often people do not initially perform an exercise frequently enough to properly learn and store the movement pattern, which results in constant difficulty with performing it properly and possibly develops faulty motor patterns that are inefficient and incur compensation.[11]

At the other end of this spectrum are those who perform an exercise far too frequently. This habit, when combined with the exclusion of alternate exercises, can create *pattern overload*, which results in development of muscular imbalances, connective tissue strain, and possible wear patterns of joint surfaces.[11]

Frequency of a routine depends on several factors, one of which is recovery. All muscles recover at different rates; larger muscles take longer than smaller ones. Fast-twitch muscles also take longer to recover than slow-twitch.[27, 28] Therefore, exercise routines that include high-intensity, low-rep training for large fast-twitch muscles should have less frequency and longer recovery time than low-intensity, high-rep training for slow-twitch muscles.

Frequency and recovery can vary due to the individual differences of each person. Some people recover faster than others and perform better with more frequency depending on their genetics, present condition, age, gender, health status, diet, and experience. Because of this, the optimal frequency of training routines is highly specialized according to the individual, the muscles trained, and the training phase and cycle.

However, despite of all these facts, unless dealing with an elite or professional athlete whose life revolves around his or her training schedule, it is often best to keep frequency of training as consistent as possible. Adherence to the program is as important as the program itself; it has been my experience that when a program requires constant changes in frequency of training, adherence is poor. It is better to stick to the most realistic frequency your life will allow. Plan for routines in need for more recovery by following them with sessions composed of more active stretching, balance, and stability work, or muscular endurance and cardiovascular training. These microcycles within a training phase help to maintain frequency and adherence, and will be covered in greater detail later in this chapter.

Recovery

Typically, recovery is the variable of program design that is least considered. The amount of recovery between workouts is set more by schedule than need or design. It is easy to get caught up in planning for all the work and totally forget about the importance of rest. Recovery is necessary for the adaptation process referred to as *supercompensation*. It might take 2 to 10 days for tissue repair and protein synthesis, depending on the levels of intensity. In other words, muscles become bigger and stronger while resting, not while training.[27]

Lack of recovery between workout routines leads to exhaustion and overtraining. *Exhaustion* is the result of short-term imbalances of stress and recovery, whereas *overtraining* is the long-term result.[38] Overtraining causes declines in tissue repair and nervous system function. It can create hormonal imbalances and often results in severe deficiencies of the immune system, leaving the person weaker, chronically fatigued, mentally drained, and prone for illness. Here, self-awareness, instinct, and common sense come into the science of program design.

At times, the body simply cannot keep pace with even the best-planned training systems, often because of the external uncontrollable variables in a person's life that gradually or suddenly add more stress to the equation than anticipated. If a person is obviously becoming ill or is experiencing a continuing or newly added stress, such as challenges at work or a marital problem, longer recovery will be needed. When these events occur and more recovery becomes necessary, try temporary reductions in training volumes and the duration of the workouts rather than decreasing the frequency of training. This will often help to maintain overall adherence to the program, and it often helps to improve recovery psychologically and physiologically.

The amount of recovery, or rest between sets, is also an important variable that is often overlooked or done totally by feel. The amount of time spent resting between a set is as important for neuromuscular adaptation as the stimulus itself. After studying the table of the neural-metabolic continuum (shown earlier in this chapter), the time required for proper recovery between sets of varying intensity and durations becomes more apparent. You will need more rest when working with higher intensity, as this type of sets requires more neural energy to stimulate maximal amounts of motor units that control the IIB fast-twitch fibers of the short-term ATP-CP energy system. Nerve cells take five to six times longer to recover than muscle cells, increasing the mandatory time to accomplish close-to-complete recovery.

However, this recovery time does not always have to be totally inactive. Active rest, such as stretching, might assist with recovery; another option is *supersetting*. Supersetting is accomplished through working opposite or unrelated muscle groups to the movement that was just completed. Supersetting allows for adequate metabolic and specific neural system recovery while continuing to train other muscles. Training routines that incorporate stretching and *supersetting* for active recovery are especially popular whenever maximal strength gains are not as high a priority as other needs or goals, such as flexibility, conditioning, or hypertrophy.

Sequence

Sequence is the specific planned exercise order in a given routine. This program variable must be planned to allow for the largest amount of random change in a training program because of the numerous uncontrollable variables that can influence exercise sequence. Being late to a training session, training at a different facility, broken or missing equipment, the presence of other people, or personal health status are just a few of the situations that can force immediate changes in the exercise sequence for that session.

However, this does not mean that the proper intensities and volumes for the planned training phase must be completely altered. It does mean that any time an exercise is moved from its originally designed sequence it will be affected, and might very well affect all following exercises to some degree. For example, consider the effects of moving a barbell squat that was planned for the first circuit in a training routine to the last circuit. Other leg movements and back exercises normally following the squat will now be easier to perform, while the squat itself will probably have to be performed with reduced loads to complete the same amount of repetitions as planned.

There are numerous guidelines in fitness literature and in practice that are extremely helpful for designing efficient sequencing of exercise routines. I will list the top seven:

1. Place exercises of high neurological challenge and demand before those of low demand, for example, a dumbbell lunge before a machine leg press.

2. Place high-priority exercises before those of lower priority, for example, train the more functional movements before machine exercises.

3. Place compound movements before isolation exercises; for example, complete a dumbbell chest press before beginning a tricep extension exercise.

4. Place new exercises in the sequence before those previously mastered, as long as this does not interfere with other guidelines.

5. Place exercises requiring high balance requirements, such as wobble board squats, before fatiguing the primary movers for that exercise.

6. Place high-intensity exercises before lower-intensity ones, for example, perform those exercises selected for application of heavy loads and multiple sets before doing supplemental work during a strength phase.

7. Place exercises targeting stabilizers such as rotator cuff and lower back exercises at the end of the routine.

Keep in mind that these are only guidelines, not rules. Experienced and advanced people with higher levels of neuromuscular efficiency can purposely go outside these guidelines to accomplish different training effects. There are valid reasons for breaking each of these guidelines for the right person and the proper goal.

The sample programs in this chapter present a system that is highly adaptable to changes in sequencing. Each routine is designed with three to four circuits grouped together, each composed of two to five exercises that are biomechanically compatible with each other. The exercises target specific areas while allowing recovery of others. The circuits themselves should be kept intact, yet each can be changed in sequence if needed or desired. The exercises within each circuit can also be moved as needed without requiring dramatic changes to the rest of the routine. Individual performance on certain exercises might be affected during these situations, but the routine should still provide for similar overall training effects.

Periodization and Progression

The key to designing successful exercise programs year-round is to develop a system that efficiently manages all program variables. This long-term planning and tracking system is what periodization is all about. Periodization, for our purposes, is defined as the planned, systematic manipulation of acute program variables. Periodization is a time-proven method of programming that has been around since the early 1950s. Much like plyometric training, the origin of periodization is credited to Russia and other Eastern Block countries. It was not a formally adopted training system in the United States until about 10 years later, after Americans witnessed the superior performances of the Russian and Eastern Block athletes in world competition.[22]

Research has confirmed periodization's potential to produce significantly better results than straight set training, or linear progression models.[22] A continual variety of training stimuli is definitely necessary to progress after initial adaptations have taken place. The neuromuscular system strives for efficiency and adapts as quickly as possible to new stimuli, but only to a certain extent before progression halts or even digresses. The accepted need for variety in training has led to a plethora of training philosophies that suggests the altering of variables based more on instinct or random selection than sound scientific rationale.

A simple review of the previous material will quickly show that maintaining the optimal relationships between all program variables is not possible through instinct or random selection. Therefore, you must develop a system to achieve consistent progression. The acceptance and use of periodization has made it much more common in professional literature and in practice.

However, the methods used for periodization vary drastically and lack any set rules. Even Kraemer provides only a vague description of periodization as "a training plan which changes your workouts at regular intervals of time" (p. 17)[22]; this description gives no stipulation on how these variables should be adjusted. However, there are common terms for the components involved in periodization and some common principles for designing periodized programs.

Program Cycles

Periodized programs are almost always divided into different cycles that last for a various amount of time and are designed to focus on certain training goals more than others. *Macrocycles* are the long-term programs most often composed of several months or an entire training year. These cycles designate the general overall goals and direct all training protocols toward the desired end result.

Macrocycles are broken into more manageable segments and smaller training programs known as *mesocycles*. Mesocycles vary according to the trainer or strength coach's training philosophies, as well as according to the needs and goals of the individual. Contemporary practices typically range anywhere from 3 to 12 weeks.[8, 22, 41] Years of practical use of periodization has led me to typically design 6–8-week mesocycles. I find it difficult to see much progress with more advanced individuals in less time, and the 10–12-week mesocycles have often proven tedious to the athlete or client, who become anxious to begin the next program.

Mesocycles direct more focus on certain training goals, such as improvement of one or two bio-motor abilities and more efficient use of specific muscle fiber types and energy systems. Yet many trainers and coaches feel it is important to provide some stimulation for all energy systems and muscle fiber types during a mesocycle for most people. This is because if an energy system is completely ignored for an 8–12-week period, a considerable amount of detraining will occur for that system and its relative use of specific muscle fibers.

Other neuromuscular benefits also may be lost if too much emphasis is placed on targeting only one specific goal. For example, if an entire 8–12-week mesocycle is spent on improving muscular endurance, strength and power will definitely decrease.[41] On the other hand, a mesocycle that improperly overemphasizes maximal strength gains can cause a drop in endurance, flexibility, and even compromise hypertrophy and stability besides possibly overstraining connective tissues and joints. To avoid de-training, each mesocycle contains certain training phases in which certain specific training goals are focused on while all others are laid to rest. The distribution and duration of these phases are dictated by the mesocycle emphasis and must correlate with the general overall goals of the macrocycle.

Training phases inside mesocycles consist of one to three weeks where the specific goals become the priority. For example, a seven-week mesocycle emphasizing hypertrophy might contain four weeks of hypertrophy work beginning with one week of endurance training, divided by a week of strength training, and capped with a week of power training. This would properly emphasize hypertrophy but should also maintain endurance and possibly still improve strength. The overall flow of any macrocycle comes right down to the yearly proportion and distribution of these training phases. Therefore, phases should be set by the mesocycle that is previously set by the macrocycle's general overall goals.

Often inside a training phase there are daily microcycles that alter the repetitions, sets, and loading schemes. These microcycles are totally dependent on the training phase yet are influenced by the overall design of the mesocycle. To demonstrate this according to the preceding example, any mesocycle spending four out of seven weeks on hypertrophy is suspect for detraining in other areas. Therefore, the use of compound sets, or drop sets, during some of these phases would be a logical choice for maintaining a certain level of muscular endurance, whereas use of pyramid loading and wave loading schemes, as well as mixing in occasional high-intensity sets and use of negative training during some of the hypertrophy routines, will maintain, or possibly improve, maximal strength. More plainly presented, it is often advantageous to occasionally perform a few low-intensity, high-rep sets and a few high-intensity, low-rep sets during long phases of hypertrophy to maintain endurance and strength benefits obtained in previous mesocycles. The following table shows the relationships of macrocycles, mesocycles, phases, and microcycles.

Periodization Cycles and Phases

Training Period	Typical Length of Time	Characteristics
Macrocycle	One training year	General plan, overall goals
Mesocycle	6–8 weeks	Detailed plan, specific goals
Training Phases	1–3 weeks	Endurance, hypertrophy, strength, power
Microcycles	Daily	Fine adjustments for maintaining goals

Training Phases

The long-term macrocycle efficiency is dependent on mesocycle program design and comes down to the proportional distribution and duration of all individual training phases. The following list presents a summary of a few optional training phases that may compose a mesocycle:

* **Transitional phase:** This phase is typically the first week of a mesocycle and is characterized by low-intensity and low-volume training. It is common to place these weeks following mesocycles that end with high-intensity strength or power phases. During this week, you should do assessments to measure progress and identify any adaptations achieved in the previous mesocycle. The new program is designed and introduced to the body with an

emphasis on training technique. You learn new movement patterns, practice the exercise sequence, and discuss diet and nutritional strategies. This phase is often termed as an active-recovery phase by many authors but it can be a very productive period as well.

* **Endurance/adaptation phase:** This phase is characterized by lower-intensity, but higher-volume routines. Muscular and cardiovascular endurance is the primary focus. However, it is also a logical phase for focusing on repetitive performance of new motor patterns, as it takes the neuromuscular system several repetitions to learn these new movements. Exercises requiring different stabilization strategies, or having high balance demands, are ideal for implementation during these phases. As seen in the neurological-metabolic continuum table earlier in this chapter, endurance training can last from 95 seconds to more than 3 minutes of time under tension. Therefore, you can use further descriptive terminology to more accurately specify the training phase. *High-intensity endurance* phases would pick up right where hypertrophy leaves off with repetitions typically set in the upper teens and lower twenties. *Low-intensity endurance* phases or sets would specify longer times under tension comprised of repetitions in the high twenties to thirties, and possibly lasting for several minutes.

* **Hypertrophy phase:** This phase is where the greatest amount of muscle hypertrophy or muscle growth occurs for most people. The overlap of increased intensity and the maintenance of high-to-moderate volume make this phase highly metabolic and induces greater hormonal responses than other training phases. Recommendations for sets and repetitions being 3–5 sets for 6–12 repetitions are typical for these phases. Because hypertrophy can overlap into other phases, we can use additional terminology to better describe the goals of the phase. *Hypertrophy-endurance* would specify higher volumes of training for greater metabolic adaptations as the goal of this phase. *Hypertrophy-strength* and *hypertrophy-power* are also common descriptions for specific training phases that would be characterized by use of higher intensities and incorporate longer rest periods and possibly include more plyometric and power movements.

Regardless of whether this is the intent, hypertrophy phases are the most commonly prescribed phases of training for general fitness. Many believe this mid-zone of training will bring them a reasonable amount of muscle growth, muscular strength, and endurance. As such, this oversimplification often leads people to training in this energy system and training phase indefinitely. As a result of constantly training in this hypertrophy zone, most individuals will experience only moderate gains toward their goals, or possibly achieve undesirable muscle mass gains. This is often the case for women who were looking for more defined musculature, but instead experienced large increases of muscle mass in the thighs and glutes due to inappropriate volumes of hypertrophy training. Although this phase might be dominant for many people according to their overall and specific training goals, it is much more effective to apply a greater variety of stimulation to the body through systematic periodization, as previously described.

* **Maximal-strength phase:** This phase is characterized by high levels of intensity and reduced volumes of work. Greater rest periods and slower training tempos to maximize motor unit recruitment are also typical of maximal-strength phases. These phases focus on more neural and intramuscular adaptations than metabolic changes desired in the hypertrophy and endurance phases. Stability is a prerequisite for maximal strength; therefore, fewer exercises and positioning options, which require high balance demands, are

selected. You can maintain these skills with occasional implementation of sets throughout the mesocycle that focus on these type of demands. Strength phases may overlap other training phases and may also incorporate other goals. *Strength-hypertrophy* phases, which vary slightly from the *hypertrophy-strength* phases mentioned previously, and *strength-power* phases are descriptive names that further specify the training phase's focus.

* **Power phases:** To produce power, the speed or rate of force production is as important, if not more so, than the amount of force produced. For this reason, power phases of training are characterized by use of moderate-intensity and even low-intensity loads, coupled with low volumes of sets and repetitions. Plyometric movements, power exercises, and medicine ball training are all common elements of a power phase. Power training has a high neural demand for the quick productions and reductions of force, plus the increased need for dynamic stability and balance. Therefore, power exercises are typically prescribed with low repetitions, moderate sets, extremely fast tempos, and sequenced early in the routine.

The integration and blending of all these various training phases of each mesocycle comprise the weekly steps toward the overall training goals of the designed macrocycle. The following figure provides an example of a macrocycle designed for a well-balanced, recreational athlete whose overall goals include increased conditioning, improved musculature, greater strength, and year-round improved performance in a variety of athletic activities. This person tapers off on activity at the end of the year so he or she can focus more on maximal strength and power gains during these later months.

Sample Yearly Macrocycle

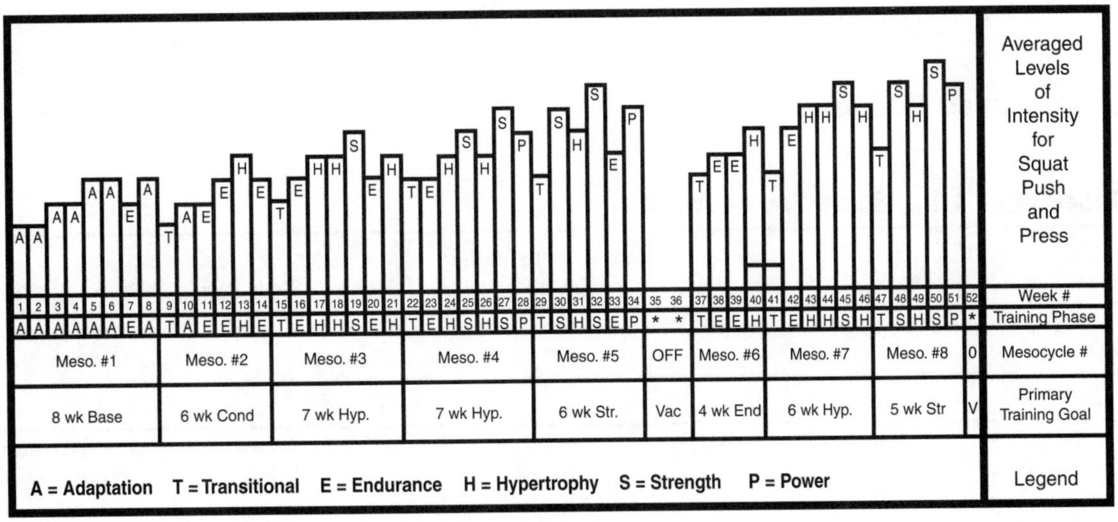

Training phase distribution of a macrocycle.

The Base Program

Each mesocycle is a miniature program in itself with the design dependent on the specific needs and goals of the individual in mind. When starting an exercise program or starting up again after a prolonged layoff, it is important that the first, and possibly the first several mesocycles are programs focused on developing a fitness base. The priorities of a base program are the development of the first four bio-motor abilities, which provide the foundation for improved performance as pictured in the first figure presented in this chapter: Increased strength and stability, adequate endurance, and joint mobility are the goals of the base program.

The needs of the individual as determined through a detailed assessment take priority over his or her individual training goals. Establishing core strength and control, joint integrity of the spine, pelvis, and shoulder girdles, attempting to correct any muscular imbalances, and strengthen all existing weak links are also primary tasks of the base program. This process will most often take more than one mesocycle to accomplish. Therefore, certain aspects of the base program will carry on into several successive mesocycles.

The following table depicts a typical base program and demonstrates the priorities of this mesocycle through the selection of the various exercises and the assignments of several program variables. Core exercises are immediately introduced and trained; then the resulting increased control is integrated into every exercise performed. It is extremely important to implement core training in the beginning; otherwise, you learn movement patterns using different stabilization strategies and breathing methods that are less harmonious with the designed function of the inner unit.

The outer trunk musculature is also targeted, and certain isolated movements for the hip and shoulder joints are common additions to a base program. Positioning options that require increased ankle, hip, and spinal stability are used along with a few balance exercises. Finally, training neuromuscular efficiency of the seven general movement patterns that have the most transfer for life and sport movements begins in a base program. You may want to refer to the figures in Chapter 1 in the section "Neuromuscular Efficiency and Motor Learning" to view these general movements.

Sample Base Routine

Mesocycle #1   Base Program A

Exercise	Reps	Sets	Tempo	Sub Totals Set/ Int. V	Rest	Body Part	Notes
Treadmill Warm-Up Gait Training	*	*	Fast Walk	10 min	*	*	Posture training, corrective training
Circuit 1							
Body Weight/ Barbell Squats	15–20	2	3221	120s–160s/ 240s–320s	*	Glutes/ Quads	Extended pause at bottom position
Dumbbell and Bench Chest Press	10–12	2	3221	80s–96s/ 160s–192s	*	Chest/ Triceps	Extended pause at bottom position
Swiss Ball Trunk Flexion	10–12	2	3132	90s–108s/ 180s–216s	60s	Abs/ Obliques	Extended pause at top position
Circuit 2							
Cable 1 Leg Hamstring Flexion	8–10	3	3132	72s–90s/ 216s–270s	*	Hams/ Glutes	Extended pause at top position
Cable 1 Arm Lat Row	10–12	3	3132	90s–108s/ 270s–324s	*	POS	Lunge position
Dumbbell 1 Leg Calf Extension	12–15	3	3122	96s–120s/ 288s–320s	60s	Calves	Balance at top position

Exercise	Reps	Sets	Tempo	Sub Totals Set/ Int. V	Rest	Body Part	Notes
Circuit 3							
Cable Overhead Rear Delt Row	10–12	3	3122	80s–96s/ 240s–288s	*	P. Delts S. Retact.	Extended pause at back position
4-Point, 2-Point Core Activation	6–8	3	1117	60s–80s/ 180s–240s	*	Inner Unit/ Core	Hold contraction 7 seconds
Dumbbell External Rotation	12–15	2	3221	96s–120s/ 192s–240s	*	Sh. Ext. Rotators	Stabilize eccentric isometric phase
Active Stretching	*	*	*	10 min	*	*	Focus on Hams., Hip Flex., Hip Int. Rotators

Mesocycle #1   Base Program B

Exercise	Reps	Sets	Tempo	Sub Totals Set/ Int. V	Rest	Body Part	Notes
Warm Up Versa Climber	*	*	*	5 min	*	POS	Focus on pulling motion
Circuit 1							
Balance Squats	15–20	2	3221	120s–160s/ 240s–320s	*	Glutes/ Quads. Add.	Frontal plane axis
Squat Rack Pushups	10–12	2	3221	80s–96s/ 160s–192s	*	Chest/ Triceps	Extended pause at bottom position
Cable Standing Hip Abduction	10–12	2	3132	90s–108s/ 180s–216s	*	Glute Med./ Abd.	Stabilize concentric isometric phase
Cable Lat Pulldown	10–12	2	3132	90s–108s/ 180s–216s	60s	Lats./ Rhom. Bi	Hold bottom position
Circuit 2							
Barbell Hip Extension	8–10	3	3221	64s–80s/ 192s–240s	*	Hams/ Glutes	Extended pause at bottom position
Dumbbell 1 Arm & 1 Leg Delt Press	10–12	2	3221	80s–96s/ 160s–192s	*	A. Delt-Tri/ LS	Balance with no external support
Cable 1 Arm Rear Delt Row	10–12	2	3122	80s–96s/ 160s–192s	*	P. Delt-Bi/ POS	Lunge position/ Hold at top
Inc. Bench, Reverse Trunk Flexion	10–12	3	3122	64s–80s/ 192s–240s	60s	Abs./ Obliques	Hold at top position
4-Point, 2-Point Core Activation	6–8	3	1117	60s–80s/ 180s–240s	*	Inner Unit/ Core	Hold contraction 7 seconds
Active Stretching	*	*	*	*	*	*	Focus on Sh. Int. Rot., Hams, Hip Ext. Rot.

Advanced Whole-Body Programs

Once a person progresses and has addressed individual needs, established core control, and developed proficiency to perform the seven general motor patterns, then more advanced routines can commence. Now, more focus on training goals begins as structural needs and health concerns have been addressed and a solid fitness base is in place. Isolated movements designed for correction of muscular imbalances are replaced with more integrated compound movements, along with a few optional isolated exercises designed for targeting specific muscles for more hypertrophy goals.

Further improvements in strength, endurance, joint balance, and advanced motor learning continue with mesocycles that contain more specific training phases and include exercise routines with more challenging combinations and sequences of exercises. Speed, agility, and power exercises are introduced in these advanced programs. The programs can be composed of whole-body routines or split routines, depending on the amount of training time available and the goals and capabilities of the individual. Considerable progression and possibly several programs are necessary between the base program example and the following advanced routines.

The routines described in the following table are examples of advanced whole-body workouts for balanced people with no particular training needs who desire overall increased fitness, some reduction of body fat, moderate gains in muscle mass, increased strength, and improved power for better athletic performance. Although both routines contain exercises to train the entire body, they each contain different movement patterns and place the body in a variety of positions while working against external loads aligned at different angles. This is done to achieve different intermuscular and intramuscular adaptations, and often to accomplish common structural needs for individuals at this level while still pursuing training goals. Varying levels of intensity and volume are offered by the different training phases that could be integrated throughout the mesocycle. This periodized approach will target different energy systems and various muscle fiber types during each individual phase as directed by the mesocycle design.

Sample Advanced Whole Body Routines

Mesocycle #3　Whole-Body A　Hypertrophy Phase

Exercise	Reps	Sets	Tempo	Sub Totals Set/ Int. V	Rest	Body Part	Notes
Warm-Up Agility Drills	5 each	*	Half Speed Full Speed	10 min	30s	*	Lateral Shuffle, Carioca, Shuttles
Circuit 1							
Barbell Squats	15–20 10–12	1 3	3121	70s–140s 350s–392s	*	Glutes/Quads	Nonlock at Top/ Constant Tempo
Dumbbell and Ball Incline Press	10–12 8–10	2	3221	80s–96s 160s–192s	*	Chest/Triceps	Extended Pause at Bottom Position
Machine Hamstring Flexion	10–12 8–10 6–8	1 1 2	3121	42s–84s 210s–266s	*	Hamstrings	Pause at Top Position
S Ball, Alternating Straight Leg Hip Flex	10–12 each	3	4221	90s–108s 270s–324s	60s	Hip Flex./ Abs. Stab.	Pause at Bottom, Ham. Active Stretch

Exercise	Reps	Sets	Tempo	Sub Totals Set/ Int. V	Rest	Body Part	Notes
Circuit 2							
Cable Standing Hip Abduction	10–12	2	2121	50s–60s 100s–120s	*	Glute Med/ Hip Abd.	Nonbraced
Cable 1 Arm Lat Row	10–12 8–10	1 2	3121	56s–84s 182s–224s	*	POS	Lunge Position
Dumbbell Single-Leg Calf Extension	10–12	3	3122	80s–96s 240s–288s	60s	Calves	Balance at Top Position
Med Ball, Single-Leg Traveling Lunges	15–17	2	2221	105s–119s 210s–238s	*	Glutes/Quads	Side Load Stabilize at Bottom
Circuit 3							
Dumbbell Shoulder Press	10–12	2	3121	70s–84s 140s–168s	*	A. Delt/ Glute-Quad	Lunge position
Dumbbell Bicep Flexion	10–12	2	3121	70s–84s 140s–168s	*	Biceps/ Glute-Quad	Lunge position
Assisted Lat Pullup	10–12	2	3121	70s–84s 140s–168s	*	Lats/Rhom. Bi	Focus on Scapular Depression and Downward Rot.
Active Stretching	*	*	*	10 min	*	*	Focus on Hams., Hip Int. Rot

Mesocycle #3   Whole-Body B   Hypertrophy Phase

Exercise	Reps	Sets	Tempo	Sub Totals Set/ Int. V	Rest	Body Part	Notes
Warm-Up Agility Drills	5 each	*	Half Speed Full Speed	10 min	30s	*	Lateral Shuffle, Carioca, Shuttles
Circuit 1							
Dumbbell Reverse Lunge	12–15	3	212.5	66s–82s 198s–246s	*	Glute-Quad/ Hip Abd.	Alternating
Dumbbell and Bench Chest Press	10–12 6–8	1 4	3121	42s–84s 238s–308s	*	Chest/ Triceps	Maximal effort
Dumbbell Wide Squat or Jump and Reach	12–15 10–12	1 3	3221	80s–120s 330s–408s	*	Glutes/ Quads	Squat-extended; pause at bottom
Assisted Overhead Lat Row-Up	8–10	4	4122	72s–90s 288s–360s	60s	Lats./P. Delt, Biceps	Pause at top
Circuit 2							
Cable Quad Extension	10–12	2	2121	50s–60s 100s–120s	*	Quad/ Hip Flex.	Active Stretching, hamstrings
Cable 1 Arm Incline Press	10–12	2	2121	50s–60s 100s–120s	*	Chest/ AOS	Lunge position
Cable Overhead Bicep Flexion	10–12	2	3122	80s–96s 240s–288s	*	Biceps/ A. Delt.	Extended hold at top position
Machine, Bent Knee Calf Extension	17–20	2	4122	153s–180s 306s–360s	60s	Glutes/ Quads	Extended hold at top position

continues

Mesocycle #3   Whole-Body B   Hypertrophy Phase *continued*

Exercise	Reps	Sets	Tempo	Sub Totals Set/ Int. V	Rest	Body Part	Notes
Circuit 3							
Cable Hamstring Flexion	10–12 8–10	1 2	3121	56s–84s 182s–224s	*	Hamstr./ Glute	Balance at top position
Cable 1 Arm Low Rear Delt Row	10–12	3	3121	70s–84s 210s–252s	*	P. Delts/ POS	Lunge position
Cable Trunk Rotation with Push or Med Ball Rotational Throw	10–12	3	2111	50s–60s 150s–180s	30s	Abs-Obliqu/ AOS	Acceleration Deceleration
Active Stretching	*	*	*	10 min	*	*	Focus on Hams., Sh. Ext. Rot., Hip Int. Rot

Advanced Split Programs

If training frequency is increased to four or more days a week, or if recovery between workouts is not adequate, performing *split programs* is the next step. Split programs utilize workout routines that emphasize certain areas of the body while avoiding unnecessary work on other areas. The subsequent routines then focus on these other areas while allowing the first areas to rest.

Split routines can divide the body from anywhere between two to five sections that are worked on using some method of alternating sequences. Five-day split programs mean that it will take five sessions to complete the training program for the entire body, whereas four-day split takes four sessions, and so on. As the neuromuscular system needs a certain amount of stimulus on a regular basis for adaptation to occur, a good rule of thumb for most goals is to train each muscle group at least twice a week.

However, since most people have definite restrictions on training frequency, I have seen a lot of success in simply dividing the body into halves and utilizing a periodized four-day split program. The program will contain two different routines for each half of the body. Training schedule is typically spread out through the week by training a couple of days in a row with a following day off, then a couple of more days in a row with another day or two off. Off days from training can include additional agility training, aerobic system training, sport-specific practices, and additional stretching routines depending on the needs and goals.

You can divide the body by observing kinetic movement, such as designing push and pull routines, or you can view it more topographically (for example, designing upper and lower body routines). The following split routines are somewhat a combination of both, and divide the body into anterior and posterior halves. Most pushing patterns will work anterior muscles, while pulling patterns will challenge posterior musculature. The glutes, which are the largest muscles on the body, receive some work on each training routine. They actually will receive more work during the anterior routines, as they are highly involved in all lower-body pushing movements such as squats, leg presses, and lunges. Also, the glutes will receive some work during poserior routines for stabilization requirement and any hip extension movements. One or two days of rest after two consecutive workdays usually provides enough recovery time for this primary muscle for most people training at this level.

These routines are presented at different points of the same mesocycle to demonstrate the numerous manipulations of acute program variables, as well as changes in exercise selection and technique. Study of these routines will show obvious variations in repetitions, sets, tempos, intensity, rest periods, and sequencing. More subtle, yet equally important, are the changes in stabilization and balance demands, use of various training tools and machines, positioning options, and technique modifications for each specific training phase, which correspond with the present goals. More speed, agility, and power movements are also added as needed to efficiently improve athletic performance. However, the basic routine and movement patterns I selected for improvement during this mesocycle remain intact.

Mesocycle #2   Anterior A   Endurance-Adaptation Phase

Exercise	Reps	Sets	Tempo	Sub Totals Set/ Int. V	Rest	Body Part	Notes
Warm-Up Agility Drills	5 each	*	Half Speed Full Speed	10 min	30s	*	Lateral Shuffle, Carioca, Shuttles
Circuit 1							
Dumbbell, Reverse Crane Lunges	15–17	3	2211	90s–102s 270s–306s	*	Glutes/ Quads	Pause at bottom/ Balance at top
Dumbbell, Delt Press	15–17	3	2121	90s–102s 270s–306s	*	A. Delt/ Glute-Quad	Lunge position
Dumbbell, Bicep Flexion	15–17	3	2121	90s–102s 270s–306s	30s	Biceps/ Glute-Quad	Lunge position
Circuit 2							
Cable, Standing 1 Arm Chest Adduction	15–17	2	3112	105s–119s 210s–238s	*	Chest/ AOS	Lunge position
Cable, Quad Extension	15–17	2	2121	90s–102s 180s–204s	*	Quad/ Hip Flexors	One arm braced
Med Ball, Pullover Throw	15	2	*	*	60s	Abs./ Obliques	Supine
Circuit 3							
Dumbbell, Wide Squats	15–17	3	2221	105s–119s 315s–357s	*	Glutes/ Quads	Extended pause at bottom position
Squat Rack, Pushup	15–17	3	3121	105s–119s 315s–357s	*	Chest/ Hip Flex	Stabilize with single leg
Swiss Ball, Leg Raise	12	2	4141	120s 240s	*	Hip Flex/ Abs Stab.	Piston movement, stabilize neck
Circuit 4							
Dumbbell, Bicep Flexion	15–17	2	2121	90s–102s 180s–204s	*	Biceps/ Glute-Quad	Lunge position
Jump Rope	*	3	*	120s–180s	60s	Calves, Quads	Feet together, single leg alt.
Active Stretching	*	*	*	10 min	*	*	Focus on Hip Flex. and Int. Rot., Sh. Int. Rot. and Pecs.

Mesocycle #2   Posterior A   Endurance-Adaptation Phase

Exercise	Reps	Sets	Tempo	Sub Totals Set/ Int. V	Rest	Body Part	Notes
Warm-Up Agility Drills	5 each	*	Half Speed Full Speed	10 min	30s	*	Backward Run, Box Drills
Circuit 1							
Dumbbell, Single-Leg Hip Extension	15–17	3	3231	135s–153s 405s–459s	*	Glutes/ Quads	Pause at bottom/ Ankle-hip stab.
Cable, 1 Arm Overhead Tricep Ext.	15–17	3	2121	90s–102s 270s–306s	*	Tricep/ AOS	Lunge position
Cable, Lat Pulldown	15–17	3	2121	90s–102s 270s–306s	30s	Lats/ Rhom. Biceps	Focus on scapular movement
Circuit 2							
Cable, Hamstring Flexion	12–15	2	3121	84s–105s 168s–210s	*	Hams/ Glutes	One arm braced
Cable, 1 Arm Lat Row	15–17	2	3122	120s–136s 240s–272s	*	Lats/ POS	Lunge position
Dumbbell, Single-Leg Calf Extension	15–17	2	2122	105s–119s 210s–238s	*	Calves	Balance at top
Cable, 1 Arm Overhead Rear Delt Row	15–17	2	2122	105s–119s 210s–238s	30s	P. Delt./ Scap. Retr.	Extended pause at back position
Circuit 3							
Machine, Hamstring Flexion	10–12	2	2122	70s–84s 140s–168s	*	Hamstrings	Extended pause at top position
Assisted, Overhead Lat Row-Up	15–17	2	2121	90s–102s 180s–204s	*	Lats/ P. Delt. Biceps	
Cable, Tricep Extension	15–17	2	2121	90s–102s 180s–204s	*	Triceps/ Scap. Dep.	Maintain optimal posture
Med Ball, Overhand Throw	12	2	*	*	30s	Spinal-Hip Extensors	
Active Stretching	*	*	*	10 min	*	*	Focus on Hamstr., Ext. Hip Rot., Lats., Tris.

Mesocycle #2   Anterior B   Endurance-Adaptation Phase

Exercise	Reps	Sets	Tempo	Sub Totals Set/ Int. V	Rest	Body Part	Notes
Warm-Up Agility Drills	5 each	*	Half Speed Full Speed	10 min	30s	*	High knees, drum majors, 8 patterns
Circuit 1							
Balance Board, Squats	15–17	3	2211	90s–102s 270s–306s	*	Glute-Quad/ Hip Add.	Pause at bottom/ Balance at top
Dumbbell and S. Ball, 1 Arm Chest Press	15–17	3	2121	90s–102s 270s–306s	*	Chest/ AOS	Maintain posture/ Stab. head
Dumbbell, Narrow Squats	15–17	3	2121	90s–102s 270s–306s	*	Glutes/ Quads	Keep knees aligned
Swiss Ball, Reverse Trunk Flexion	12–15	3	3112	84s–105s 252s–315s	30s	Abs./ Obliques	Slight incline position

Exercise	Reps	Sets	Tempo	Sub Totals Set/ Int. V	Rest	Body Part	Notes
Circuit 2							
Med Ball, Traveling Lunge	12–15	2	3221	96s–120s 192s–240s	*	Glute-Quad/ Hip Abd.	Side load
Cable, 1 Arm Chest Press	15–17	2	2121	90s–102s 180s–204s	*	Chest/ AOS	Lunge position
Dumbbell, Bicep Flexion	15–17	2	3121	84s–105s 168s–210s	*	Biceps/ Glute-Quad	Lunge position/ Piston movement
Cable, Trunk Rotation with Push	15–17	2	2121	90s–102s 180s–204s	30s	AOS/ Glute-Quads	Lunge position
Circuit 3							
Squat Rack, Pushup	15–17	2	3221	96s–120s 192s–240s	*	Chest/ Hip Flexors	Stabilize with one leg
High Knees	*	2	*	45s–60s 90s–120s	*	Hip-Sh. Flex. Hip-Ankle Ext.	Run in place
Cable, Overhead Bicep Flexion	15–17	2	2122	84s–105s 168s–210s	30s	Biceps/ A. Delts	Hold top position
Active Stretching	*	*	*	10 min	*	*	Focus on Hip Flex. and Int. Rot., Sh. Int. Rot. and Pecs.

Mesocycle #2   Posterior B   Endurance-Adaptation Phase

Exercise	Reps	Sets	Tempo	Sub Totals Set/ Int. V	Rest	Body Part	Notes
Warm-Up Agility Drills	5 each	*	Half Speed Full Speed	10 min	30s	*	Backward Run, Backward Plant, X
Circuit 1							
Dumbbell, 1 Arm Lat Row	15–17	3	2122	105s–119s 315s–357s	*	Lats/ POS	Lunge position no brace
Machine, Single-Leg Hamstring Flexion	10–12	3	3122	80s–96s 240s–288s	*	Hamstrings	Plate load machine
Dumbbell, Single-Leg Calf Extension	15–17	3	2122	105s–119s 315s–357s	30s	Calves	Balance at top
Circuit 2							
Assisted, Lat Pullup	15–17	2	3121	105s–119s 210s–238s	*	Lats/ Rhom. Bi	Focus on scapular motion
Barbell, Hip Extension	12–15	2	2221	84s–105s 168s–210s	*	Glute-Ham/ DLS	Pause at bottom
Cable, Overhead Rear Delt Row	15–17	2	2122	105s–119s 210s–238s	*	P. Delts/ Scap Retr.	Hold back position
Swiss Ball, Tricep Extension	15–17	2	2121	75s–85s 150s–170s	30s	Triceps/ Hip Ext.	Piston movement stabilize head
Circuit 3							
Dumbbell, Rear Delt Rows	15–17	2	2122	105s–119s 210s–238s	*	P. Delt-Scap./ Hip Ext.	Hold up position
Squat Rack, Tricep Pushups	15–17	2	2121	75s–85s 150s–170s	*	Triceps/ Hip Flex Abs	*

continues

Mesocycle #2   Posterior B   Endurance-Adaptation Phase *continued*

Exercise	Reps	Sets	Tempo	Sub Totals Set/ Int. V	Rest	Body Part	Notes
Machine, Bent Leg Calf Extension	17–20	2	2122	119s–140s 238s–280s	*	Soleus	Add one set of Tibialis Flexion
Cable, Tricep Extensions	15–17	2	2121	75s–85s 150s–170s	30s	Triceps/ Scap dep.	Maintain posture
Active Stretching	*	*	*	10 min	*	*	Focus on Hamstr., Hip Ext. Rot., Lats., Tris.

Mesocycle #2   Anterior A   Hypertrophy Phase

Exercise	Reps	Sets	Tempo	Sub Totals Set/ Int. V	Rest	Body Part	Notes
Warm-Up Agility Drills	5 each	*	Half Speed/ Full Speed	10 min	30s	*	High kness, bounding
Circuit 1							
Dumbbell, Reverse Crane Lunges	10–12	4	3121	70s–84s 280s–336s	*	Glutes/ Quads	Pause at bottom/ balance at top
Dumbbell, Delt Press	8–10	4	3121	56s–70s 224s–280s	*	A. Delt/ Glute.-Quad	Lunge position
Dumbbell, Bicep Flexion	10–12	4	3121	70s–84s 280s–336s	60s	Biceps/ Glute-Quad	Lunge position
Circuit 2							
Cable, Standing Chest Adduction	8–10	4	3122	64s–80s 256s–320s	*	Chest/ AOS	Lunge position
Cable, Quad Extension	10–12	2	3121	70s–84s 140s–168s	*	Quad/ Hip Flexors	Two arms braced
Swiss Ball, Reverse Trunk Flexion	10–12	3	3121	70s–84s 140s–168s	60s	Abs./ Obliques	Inclined
Circuit 3							
Dumbbell, Wide Squats	10–12	3	3121	70s–84s 140s–168s	*	Glutes/ Quads	Pause at bottom position
Squat Rack, Pushup	15–17	2	3121	105s–119s 210s–238s	*	Chest/ Hip Flex	Stabilize with single leg
Incline Bench, Double Leg Raise	8–10	2	3121	56s–70s 112s–140s	*	Hip Flex/ Abs Stab.	Both legs
Dumbbell, Bicep Flexion	10–12	2	3121	70s–84s 140s–168s	60s	Biceps/ Glute-Quad	Symmetrical stance
Active Stretching	*	*	*	10 min	*	*	Focus on Hip Flex. and Int. Rot., Sh. Int. Rot. and Pecs.

Mesocycle #2 Posterior A Hypertrophy Phase

Exercise	Reps	Sets	Tempo	Sub Totals Set/ Int. V	Rest	Body Part	Notes
Warm-Up Agility Drills	5 each	*	Half Speed Full Speed	10 min	30s	*	Backward run-plant, shuttle runs
Circuit 1							
Barbell, Hip Extension	10–12	3	3231	90–108s 270s–324s	*	Glutes/ Quads	Extended pause at bottom position
Cable, Overhead Tri Extension	10–12	3	3121	70s–84s 210s–252s	*	Tricep/ Abs.	Lunge position
Cable, Lat. Pulldown	10–12	3	3121	70s–84s 210s–252s	60s	Lats/ Hom. Bi	Focus on scapular movement
Circuit 2							
Cable, Hamstring Flexion	8–10	3	3121	84s–105s 168s–210s	*	Hams/ Glutes	One-arm braced
Cable, 1 Arm Lat Row	8–10	3	3122	64s–80s 192s–240s	*	Lats/ POS	Lunge position
Machine, Calf Extension	10–12	3	3122	80s–96s 240s–288s	*	Calves	Extended pause at top position
Cable, Overhead Rear Delt Row	10–12	3	3122	80s–96s 240s–288s	60s	P. Delt./ Scap Retr.	Extended pause at back position
Circuit 3							
Machine, Hamstring Flexion	6–8	3	3122	48s–64s 144s–192s	*	Hamstrings	Extended pause at top position
Assisted, Overhead Lat Row-Up	8–10	2	3121	56s–70s 112s–140s	*	Lats/ P. Delt. Bi	Lean back to decrease bi. asst.
Cable, Tricep Extension	8–10	2	3121	56s–70s 112s–140s	*	Triceps/ Scap Dep.	Keep shoulder blades down
Med Ball, Forward Overhead Throw	8–10	2	*	*	30s	Lats	Downward slam
Active Stretching	*	*	*	10 min	*	*	Focus on Hamstr., Hip Ext. Rot., Lats., Tris.

Mesocycle #2 Anterior B Hypertrophy Phase

Exercise	Reps	Sets	Tempo	Sub Totals Set/ Int. V	Rest	Body Part	Notes
Warm-Up Agility Drills	5 each	*	Half Speed Full Speed	10 min	30s	*	High knees, Drum majors, 8 pattern
Circuit 1							
Barbell, Squats	20–15- 10-10-10	5	3121	70s–140s 455s	*	Glute-Quad.	Pause at bottom position
Dumbbell and Bench, Chest Press	15–10- 6–6–10	5	3121	42s–105s 329s	*	Chest/ Triceps	Modified pyramid loading
Dumbbell, Narrow Squats	Skip	*	*	*	*	*	*
Swiss Ball, Reverse Trunk Flexion	8–10	5	3122	64s–80s 192s–240s	120s	Abs./ Obliques	Hold top position

Mesocycle #2   Anterior B   Hypertrophy Phase   *continued*

Exercise	Reps	Sets	Tempo	Sub Totals Set/ Int. V	Rest	Body Part	Notes
Circuit 2							
Machine, Leg Press	20–15–10	3	3122	80s–160s 360s	*	Glute-Quad/ Hip Abd.	Hip-width foot position
Cable, 1 Arm Incline Press	8–10	3	3121	56s–70s 168s–210s	*	Chest/ AOS	Lunge position
Dumbbell, Bicep Flexion	8–10	3	3121	56s–70s 168s–210s	*	Biceps/ Glute-Quad	Lunge position/ Double-single
Cable, Trunk Rotation with Push	10–12	2	3121	70s–84s 140s–168s	60s	AOS/ Glute-quads	1st and 3rd sets
Machine, Trunk Rotation	10–12	1	2122	96s–120s 96s–120s	60s	Chest/ Hip Flexors	2nd and 4th sets
Circuit 3							
Bounding	10 each	2 × 2	*	*	*	Hip-Sh. Flex/ Hip-Ankle Ext.	Across gym floor
Cable, Overhead Bicep Flexion	8–10	2	3121	56s–70s 112s–140s	30s	Biceps/ A. Delts	Hold top position
Active Stretching	*	*	*	10 min	*	*	Focus on Hip Flex. and Int. Rot., Sh. Int. Rot. and Pecs.

Mesocycle #2   Posterior B   Hypertrophy Phase

Exercise	Reps	Sets	Tempo	Sub Totals Set/ Int. V	Rest	Body Part	Notes
Warm-Up Agility Drills	10 each	*	Half Speed Full Speed	10 min	30s	*	Diagonal running, forward and back
Circuit 1							
Barbell, Lat Row	8–10	4	3121	56s–70s 224s–280s	*	Lats/ Rhom. Bi	Narrow stance
Machine, Hamstring Flexion	10–8–6–6	4	3122	48s–80s 240s	*	Hamstrings	Hold at top position
Machine, Calf Extension	10–12	3	2122	105s–119s 315s–357s	*	Calves	Hold at top position
Machine, Bent Knee Calf Extension	17–20	3	2122	119s–140s 357s–420s	30s	Soleus	Hold at top position
Circuit 2							
Assisted, Lat Pullup	8–10	3	3121	56s–70s 168s–210s	*	Lats/ Rhom. Bi	Focus on scapular motion
Barbell and Swiss Ball, Incline Tri Extension	8–10	3	3121	56s–70s 168s–210s	*	Triceps/ Hip Ext.	
Cable, Overhead Rear Delt Row	10–12	3	3122	80s–96s 240s–288s	*	P. Delts/ Scap. Retr.	Hold back position
Cable, Hip Abduction	10–12	3	3121	70s–84s 210s–252s	*	Glute Med./ TFL	Lowest setting

Exercise	Reps	Sets	Tempo	Sub Totals Set/ Int. V	Rest	Body Part	Notes
Circuit 3							
Dumbbell, Rear Delt Rows	8–10	2	3122	80s–96s 240s–288s	*	P. Delt-Scap/ Hip Ext.	Hold up position
Med Ball, Backward Underhand Throw	10–12	2	*	*	60s	Hip Ext./ Sh. Flex.	Turn and catch
Squat Rack, Tricep Pushups	10–12	2	3121	70s–84s 140s–168s	*	Triceps/ Hip Flex. Abs	Lowest setting
Active Stretching	*	*	*	10 min	*	*	Focus on Hamstr., Hip Ext. Rot., Lats., Tris.

Mesocycle #2   Anterior A   Strength-Power Phase

Exercise	Reps	Sets	Tempo	Sub Totals Set/ Int. V	Rest	Body Part	Notes
Warm-Up Agility Drills	3 each	*	Half Speed Full Speed	5 min	30s	*	High knees, bounding
Circuit 1							
Lunge Jump	6–8	5	*	*	30s	Glutes/ Quads	As high and fast as possible
Plyo-Pushup	10–12	5	*	*	30s	Chest/ A. Delt., Triceps	A high and fast as possible
Dumbbell, Seated Bicep Flexion	6–8	5	4131	54s–72s 270s–360s	120s	Biceps	Seated with no back rest
Circuit 2							
Barbell and Bench, Incline Press	6–8	4	4122	54s–72s 216s–288s	*	Chest/ A. Delt, Triceps	*
Machine, Quad Extension	10–12	4	4121	80s–96s 320s–384s	*	Quad/ Hip Flexors	*
Swiss Ball, Reverse Trunk Flexion	6–8	4	4121	48s–64s 192s–256s	*	Abs./ Obliques	High inclined position
Dumbbell, Wide Squats	6–8	4	4121	48s–64s 192s–256s	120s	Glutes/ Quads	*
Active Stretching	*	*	*	10 min	*	*	Focus on Hip Flex. and Int. Rot., Sh. Int. Rot. and Pecs.

Mesocycle #2   Posterior A   Strength-Power Phase

Exercise	Reps	Sets	Tempo	Sub Totals Set/ Int. V	Rest	Body Part	Notes
Warm-Up Agility Drills	5 each	*	Half Speed Full Speed	5 min	30s	*	Backward run-plant, shuttle runs
Circuit 1							
Barbell, Power Clean/ Hang Clean	6–8	5 - (3 & 2)	*	*	*	Glute-Quad/ Sh.-Trap	Extended pause at bottom position
Jump and Glute Kick	8–10	5	*	*	*	Glute-Quad/ Hamstring	As high and fast as possible
Cable, Lat. Pulldown	8-6- 4-4-4	5	3131	32s–64s 208s	120s	Lats/ Rhom. Biceps	Focus on scapular movement
Circuit 2							
Barbell, Hip Extension	6–8	3	4122	54s–72s 162s–216s	*	Glutes/ Quads	Slow eccentric movement
Cable, Seated Lat Row	6–8	3	4122	54s–72s 162s–216s	*	Lats/ Rhom. Biceps	Focus on scapular movement
Barbell and Bench, Tricep Extensions	6–8	3	4122	54s–72s 162s–216s	*	Tricep	Slight decline position
Machine, Hamstring Flexion	8-6- 4-4	4	4122	36s–72s 198s	*	Hamstrings	Extended pause at top position
Circuit 3							
Med Ball, Forward Overhand Throw	8–10	4	*	*	30s	Lats	Downward slam
Active Stretching	*	*	*	10 min	*	*	Focus on Hamstr., Hip Ext. Rot., Lats., Tris.

Mesocycle #2   Anterior B   Strength-Power Phase

Exercise	Reps	Sets	Tempo	Sub Totals Set/ Int. V	Rest	Body Part	Notes
Warm-Up Agility Drills	5 each	*	Half Speed Full Speed	5 min	30s	*	High knees, drum majors
Circuit 1							
Barbell, Squats	15–10–8- 6-6-6	6	4131	54s–135s 459s	60s	Glute-Quad.	Pause at bottom position
Dumbbell and Bench Chest Press	10–6–4- 4-4-4	6	3121	28s–70s 224s	*	Chest/ Triceps	Modified pyramid loading
Swiss Ball, Double Straight Leg Raise	6–8	5	4131	54s–72s 270s–360s	*	Hip Flexors/ Abs	Slow eccentric
Swiss Ball, Reverse Trunk Flexion	6–8	5	4122	54s–72s 270s–360s	180s	Abs/ Obliques	Hold top position
Circuit 2							
Barbell, Push-Press	6–8	3	*	*	*	Glute-Quad/ Shoulders	High speed, moderate weight
Machine, Leg Press	10–8–6	3	4232	66s–10s 264s	*	Glutes/ Quads	Hip-width foot position

Exercise	Reps	Sets	Tempo	Sub Totals Set/ Int. V	Rest	Body Part	Notes
Dumbbell, Bicep Flexion	6–8	3	4121	48s–64s 144s–192s	*	Biceps/ A. Delts	Seated with back rest
Med Ball, Rotational Throw	8–10	3	*	*	120s	Obliques, LS, AOS	As fast and hard as possible
Active Stretching	*	*	*	10 min	*	*	Focus on Hip Flex. and Int. Rot., Sh. Int. Rot. and Pecs.

Mesocycle #2   Posterior B   Strength-Power Phase

Exercise	Reps	Sets	Tempo	Sub Totals Set/ Int. V	Rest	Body Part	Notes
Warm-Up Agility Drills	5 each	*	Half Speed Full Speed	5 min	30s	*	Diagonal running, forward and back
Circuit 1							
Barbell, Lat. Row	4–6	5	4121	32s–48s 160s–240s	*	Lats/ Rhom. Biceps	Narrow stance
Machine, Hamstring Flexion	8-6-4-4-4	5	4122	36s–72s 234s	*	Hamstrings	Hold at top position
Machine, Calf Extension	8–10	4	4122	72s–90s 288s–360s	*	Calves	Hold at top position
Circuit 2							
Machine, Bent Knee Calf Extension	15–17	4	4122	135s–153s 540s–612s	120s	Soleus	Hold at top position
Assisted, Lat. Pullup	6–8	4	4121	48s–64s 192s–256s	*	Lats/ Rhom. Bi	Focus on scapular motion
Barbell and Bench, Incline Tricep Ext.	6–8	4	4121	48s–64s 192s–256s	*	Triceps	Inclined position
Cable, Overhead Rear Delt Row	6–8	4	4122	54s–72s 216s–288s	*	P.Delts/ Scap Retr	Hold back position
Med Ball, Backward Underhand Throw	8–10	4	*	*	*	Hip Ext./ Trunk Ext.	Backward slam
Active Stretching	*	*	*	10 min	*	*	Focus on Hamstr., Hip Ext. Rot., Lats., Tris.

Recommendations for Periodization

When beginning periodization, remember that you must pre-establish a good fitness base with structural and health needs already addressed. You should also have experience with advanced whole-body and split programs before integrating these more structured periodized mesocycles. Once periodization begins, simply start one step at a time. Planned systematic periodization models are not mastered overnight. Begin by designing mesocycles that incorporate a few different training phases and contain a few corresponding planned changes at each phase.

Keep the routines themselves intact with only minor changes in sequence as needed for the training phase or for any uncontrollable variables. Track all changes and progress slowly, then gradually learn to coordinate other changes that would also be appropriate for the specific training phase. Try to adhere to the plan as closely as possible. Too much variation and random changes can supply an overabundance of information and stresses for the neuromuscular system to adapt to, and can be as inefficient as no variation at all. Consider these 12 tips on periodization:

1. Break macrocycles into smaller manageable programs or mesocycles.
2. Design each mesocycle with a certain amount of the various endurance, hypertrophy, strength, and power phases depending on specific training goals.
3. Begin each mesocycle with a transitional phase.
4. Practice movements and integrate positioning options that require more stabilization and balance demands while intensity is low.
5. Keep volume high while intensity is low.
6. When adding intensity, adjust volume appropriately.
7. When decreasing repetitions, increase sets and rest periods, and select fewer movements for each muscle group.
8. Make small adjustments to sequence according to the priorities of the training phase.
9. Utilize more stabilized positioning choices during phases in which you desire increased motor unit recruitment and maximal strength.
10. Decrease external loads when you desire increased speed and power, and incorporate more plyometric-type exercises.
11. Never compromise structural integrity and overall health needs for the pursuit of specific training goals.
12. Always integrate and adhere to all elements of proper exercise technique. *What* is done, can only be as efficient as *how* it is done.

Summary

Program design is a scientific process of developing systems that progress and vary training stimuli in appropriate amounts to continue beneficial adaptations for addressing needs and obtaining overall goals. There are several variables and their associated components that can be adjusted for achieving these purposes, such as intensity, volume, recovery, and sequence.

Intensity represents the amount of resistance that is used and is probably the most important variable to consider. Any changes in intensity will affect all other training variables and in a large part, determine the specific adaptations that will be experienced by the neuromuscular system. Greater internal forces must be generated in order to overcome greater intensity levels that will ultimately increase compressive and shearing forces at the joint whether this is the intent or not. These are just a few reasons that changes of intensity should always be done in a planned systematic manner.

Volume is the total amount of time under tension. Initial volume is composed of the total amount of sets, repetitions, and the tempo of each repetition that is done for a muscle group in a single routine. Total volume is the initial volume multiplied by the frequency of training sessions for the specific duration of the meso- or macrocycle. The science of selecting repetitions, sets, tempos, and frequency of training is directly related to the benefits desired from the neural-metabolic continuum of neuromuscular adaptation. Volume has interdependent relationships with intensity and recovery that requires several adjustments of its varying components to target specific energy systems and muscle fiber types. Recovery is often an overlooked variable in this process that can affect the overall adaptations experienced.

Periodization is the planned, systematic manipulation of acute program variables. This process of progressive program development can only begin after a solid fitness base has been established. Long-term planning for periodized programs includes designing macrocycles, which are often year-long plans that identify general overall goals and set a schedule for accomplishing them. Macrocycles are broken up into smaller mesocycles, which are typically 6- to 12-week programs designed to accomplish certain steps of the overall goals. Mesocycles contain several different phases where more specific goals such as endurance, hypertrophy, strength, and power become the primary focus during these weekly intervals. Proper periodization ensures that balanced training throughout the year is achieved so that all needs are addressed while overall goals are being accomplished.

I hope this book is valuable as a continued resource for your pursuit of better health and greater physical performance. By learning and following the training principles and exercise techniques presented in this book, you should not only become stronger, faster, and more powerful, but also more stable, mobile, agile, and better conditioned. Remember: It is great to train hard, but always train smart.

1. Aaberg, E. 1999. *Muscle Mechanics*. Champaign, IL: Human Kinetics.

2. ———. 2000. *Resistance Training Instruction*. Champaign, IL: Human Kinetics.

3. ———. 2001. *Resistance Training Instruction, Video Series: The Trunk*. Champaign, IL: Human Kinetics.

4. ———. 2001. *Resistance Training Instruction, Video Series: The Lower Body*. Champaign, IL: Human Kinetics.

5. ———. 2001. *Resistance Training Instruction, Video Series: The Upper Body*. Champaign, IL: Human Kinetics.

6. Alter, M. 1988, 1996. *Science of Flexibility, Second Edition*. Champaign, IL: Human Kinetics.

7. Baechle, T. National Strength and Conditioning Association. 1994. *Essentials of Strength and Conditioning*. Champaign, IL: Human Kinetics.

8. Bompa, T., and Cornacchia. 1998. *Serious Strength Training*. Champaign, IL: Human Kinetics.

9. Brown, L., V. Ferrigno, and J.C. Santana. 2000. *Training for Speed, Agility, and Quickness*. Champaign, IL: Human Kinetics.

10. Calais-Germain, B. 1993. *Anatomy of Movement*. Seattle, WA: Eastland Press.

11. Chek, P. 2000. *Movement That Matters*. Encinitas, CA: C.H.E.K. Institute.

12. ———. 1999. *The Inner Unit and the Outer Units*. ptonthenet.com: Personal Training on the Net.

13. ———. 1998. *Golf Conditioning*. Encinitas, CA: C.H.E.K. Institute.

14. ———. 1992, 1998. *Scientific Core Training, Video and Correspondence Course*. Encinitas, CA: C.H.E.K. Institute.

15. ———. 1995. *Scientific Back Training*, Encinitas, CA: C.H.E.K. Institute.

16. ———. 1995. *Program Design*. Encinitas, CA: C.H.E.K. Institute.

17. ———. 1996. *Dynamic Medicine Ball Training, Video and Correspondence Course*. Encinitas, CA: C.H.E.K. Institute.

18. Chu, D. 1992. *Jumping into Plyometrics*. Champaign, IL: Leisure Press.

19. Clark, M. 2001. *Integrated Training for the New Millennium*. Thousand Oaks, CA: National Academy of Sports Medicine.

20. Enoka, R. 1988, 1994, 2002. *Neuromechanics of Human Movement, Third Edition*. Champaign, IL: Human Kinetics.

21. Fleck, S., and W. Kraemer. 1987, 1997. *Designing Resistance Training Programs, Second Edition*. Champaign, IL: Human Kinetics.

22. ———. 1996. *Periodization Breakthrough*. Ronkonkoma, N.Y.: Advanced Research Press.

23. Foran, B. 2001. *High-Performance Sports Conditioning*. Champaign, IL: Human Kinetics.

24. Heyward, V. 1998. *Advanced Fitness Assessment and Exercise Prescription, Third Edition*. Champaign, IL: Human Kinetics.

25. Lephart, S., and F. Fu. 2000. *Proprioception and Neuromuscular Control in Joint Stability*. Champaign, IL: Human Kinetics.

26. Norkin, C., and P. Levangie. 1992. *Joint Structure and Function: A Comprehensive Analysis*. Philadelphia, PA: F.A. Davis Company.

27. Poliquin, C. 1997. *The Poliquin Principles*. Napa, CA: Dayton Writers Group.

28. ———. 1998. *Charles Poliquin's Advanced Strength Training Certification Program*. Manual Napa, CA: Dayton Publications.

29. Purvis, T. 1997. *Resistance Training Specialist, The Mastery Course Manual #1*. Oklahoma City, OK: Focus on Fitness Productions.

30. ———. 1997. *Resistance Training Specialist, The Mastery Course Manual #2*. Oklahoma City, OK: Focus on Fitness Productions.

31. ———. 1997. *Resistance Training Specialist, The Mastery Course Manual #3*. Oklahoma City, OK: Focus on Fitness Productions.

32. ———. 1997. *Resistance Training Specialist, The Mastery Course Manual #4*. Oklahoma City, OK: Focus on Fitness Productions.

33. ———. 1995. *Focus on Fitness: Instructor Video Series*. Oklahoma City, OK: Focus on Fitness Productions.

34. Radcliffe, J., and R. Farentinos. 1999. *High-Powered Plyometrics*. Champaign, IL: Human Kinetics.

35. Renstrom, P.A.F.H. 1993. *Sports Injuries: Basic Principles of Prevention and Care.* Osney, Mead, Oxford: Blackwell Scientific Publications.

36. Richardson, C., G. Jull, P. Hodges, and J. Hides. 1999. *Therapeutic Exercise for Spinal Segmental Stabilization in Low Back Pain.* London: Churchill Livingstone of Harcourt Publishers Limited.

37. Schmidt, R.H. 1991. *Motor Learning and Performance.* Champaign, IL: Human Kinetics.

38. Siff, M. 2000. *Supertraining, Fifth Edition.* Denver, CO: M. Siff. Supertraining Institute.

39. ————. 1998. *Facts and Fallacies of Fitness*, Second Edition. Johannesburg, South Africa: M. Siff.

40. Vleeming, A., V. Mooney, T. Dorman, C. Snijders, and R. Stoeckart. 1997. *Movement, Stability and Low Back Pain.* New York, NY: Churchill Livingstone.

41. Ward, P., and R. Ward. 1997. *The Encyclopedia of Weight Training, Second Edition.* Laguna Hills, CA. QPT Publications.

42. Watkins, J. 1999. *Structure and Function of the Musculoskeletal System.* Champaign, IL: Human Kinetics.

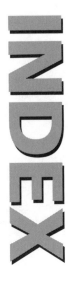

INDEX

A

absolute-strength, 35
acceleration-strength, 35, 48
actin (contractile protein filament), 7
active flexibility, 40
active insufficiency (muscles), 9
active stretching, 42
active system (movement), 1, 6-10, 17-24
adaptation to time under tension, neural-metabolic continuum, 188
advanced split programs, 202-210
advanced whole-body programs, 199-200
agility, 51
  exercises
    backpedal plants with sprint, 170
    backpedaling, 170
    bounding, 167
    carioca, 169
    drum majors, 167
    figure eight pattern, 172
    glute kickers, 166
    high knees, 166
    lateral crossover run, 169
    lateral shuffle, 168
    power skipping, 168
    shuttle run patterns, 172
    square pattern, 171
    X pattern, 171
  improving, 50-52
  neuromuscular coordination, 51
  SAID Principle, 53
  speed training, 52
  training, 53
agonists (muscles), 17
alignment, resistance training, 66-67
alpha neurons, spinal cord, 25
amortization phase (power), 54
anaerobic threshold, 37
antagonists (muscles), 17
anterior motor neurons (spinal cord), 25
anterior oblique subsystem (AOS), 134
  muscles, 23
AOS (anterior oblique subsystem), muscles, 23
aponeurosis tendon, 20
appendicular skeleton, 3
articular cartilage, 6
assignments, tempo, 73-74
associated control (coordination), 51
autonomous control (coordination), 51
axial skeleton, 3

B

backpedal plants with sprint exercise, 170
backpedaling exercise, 170
backward underhand throw (med ball) exercise, 180
balance
  reflexes, 39
    body-righting, 39
    tilting-response, 39
  resistance training, 71
balance squats, 108
barbell exercises
  chest press, 132
  dead-lift, 112
  hip extensions, 103
  lat roll, 139
  scapular elevation, 149
  squats, 111
  triceps press, 159
base program, training, 197-198
bench exercises
  chest press, 132
  incline press, 135
  triceps press, 159
biaxial joints, 5
bio-motor abilities, 45, 184
  agility, improving, 50-52
  endurance, improving, 36-38
  improving, 33
  mobility, improving, 39-43
  power, improving, 52-55
  speed, improving, 46-50
  stability, improving, 38-39
  strength, improving, 33-36
body-righting reflexes, 39, 71
body weight exercises
  reverse lunge, 116
  stationary lunge, 114

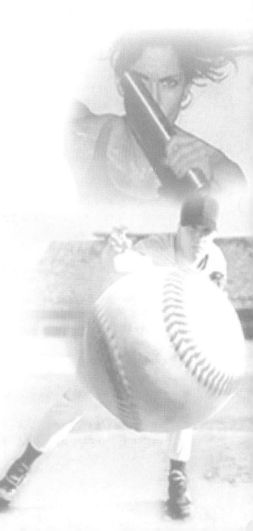

bones
    groups of, 3
    joints, 3, 5
        connective tissue, 5-6
        isolated joint kinematics, 9-10
bounding exercise, 167
brain
    cerebral cortex, 28
    lower, 26-27
brain stem, 26
breathing, exercise, 74-76

C

cable exercises
    ham flexion, 123
    hip abduction, 105-106
    one-arm bicep flexion, 163
    one-arm decline press (lunge press), 134
    one-arm low lat row, 143
    one-arm low rear delt row, 148
    one-arm triceps extension, 158
    overhead bicep flexion, 162
    overhead lat row, 142
    overhead rear delt row, 147
    overhead triceps extension, 157
    quad extensions, 121
    seated lat pulldown, 144
    seated lat row, 141
    shoulder horizontal external rotation, 152
    shoulder horizontal internal rotation, 153
    shoulder integrated external rotation, 154
    shoulder integrated internal rotation, 155
capsules (joints), 6
carioca exercise, 169
cartilage, 6
cartilaginous joints, 5
caudate nucleus, 28
cerebellum, 27
cerebral cortex, 28
cognitive control (coordination), 51
concentric contractions (muscles), 9
connective tissue, joints, 5-6
contract-contract stretching, 42

control system (movement), 1, 24-30
coordination, agility, 51
core control (strength), 53
core function, stabilization, 72
curvilinear motion, resistance training, 61

D

deep longitudinal subsystem (DLS), 21-22
deficits, flexibility, 40
DLS (deep longitudinal subsystem), 21-22
drum majors exercise, 167
dumbbell exercises
    bicep flexion, 161
    chest press, 130
    delt press (lunge press), 137
    incline press, 135
    narrow squats, 110
    one-arm and -leg delt press, 138
    one-arm chest press, 131-132
    one-arm incline press, 136
    one-arm lat row, 140
    one-leg calf extension, 125
    one-leg hip extension, 104
    rear delt row, 146
    reverse lunge, 117
    shoulder external rotation, 150
    shoulder internal rotation, 151
    stationary lunge, 115
    traveling lunge, 119
    triceps extension, 156
    wide squats, 109
dynamic endurance strength, 35
dynamic stability, 38, 70

E

eccentric contraction (muscles), 9
endomysium (protective fascia, muscle fibers), 7
endurance
    anaerobic threshold, 37
    improving, 36-38
    local muscular endurance, 36
    maximal oxygen consumption (VO2 max), 36
    OBLA (onset of blood lactate accumulation), 37

    speed, 53
    strength, 53
endurance-strength, 35
epimysium, 7
exercise breathing, science of, 75
exercise motion, resistance training, 60-66
    path of motion, 60-61
    range of motion, 61-65
    type of motion, 60-61
exercises
    backpedal plants with sprints, 170
    backpedaling, 170
    backward underhand throw (med ball), 180
    bounding, 167
    carioca, 169
    drum majors, 167
    figure eight pattern, 172
    forward overhand throw (med ball), 179
    forward pass (med ball), 178
    forward pullover throw (med ball), 179
    forward underhand throw (med ball), 178
    glute kickers, 166
    hang clean, 181
    hexagon jump pattern, 177
    high knees, 166
    jump and reach, 173
    jump and tuck, 173
    jump with glute kick, 174
    lateral crossover run, 169
    lateral jumps, 176
    lateral shuffle, 168
    lateral throw (med ball), 180
    long jumps (hops), 175
    lower body exercises
        balance squats, 108
        barbell dead-lift, 112
        barbell hip extension, 103
        barbell squats, 111
        body weight squats, 107
        body weight, reverse lunge, 116
        body weight, stationary lunge, 114
        cable hip abduction, 105
        cable hip adduction, 106
        cable, ham flexion, 123
        cable, quad extension, 121

dumbbell wide squats, 109

dumbbell, narrow squats, 110

dumbbell, one-leg calf extension, 125

dumbbell, one-leg hip extension, 104

dumbbell, reverse lunge, 117

dumbbell, stationary lunge, 115

dumbbell, traveling lunge, 119

flat bench, bent-leg hip flexion, 98

forty-five degree hip extension, 102

incline bench, straight-leg hip flexion, 99

inclined bench, double-leg hip extension, 101

iso-kinetic tib flexion, 129

machine, bent-leg calf extension, 127

machine, calf extension, 126

machine, ham flexion, 124

machine, quad extension, 122

machine, seated leg lift, 113

machine, tib flexion, 128

med ball, traveling lunge (side load), 120

Swiss ball, double-leg hip flexion, 100

traveling lunge, 118

lunge jump, 175

power clean, 181

power pushups, 182

power skipping, 168

push-press (jerk), 182

reverse trunk exercises

incline bench, trunk extension, 91

Swiss ball, reverse trunk flexion, 90

Swiss ball, trunk extension, 92

shuttle run patterns, 172

single-leg lateral jumps, 177

square pattern, 171

stabilization, 79

four-point core activation, 80

one-point core activation, 84

quadroplex, 82

standing core activation, 83

supine core activation, 85-86

two-point core activation, 81

strength, 79

four-point core activation, 80

one-point core activation, 84

quadraplex, 82

standing core activation, 83

supine core activation, 85-86

two-point core activation, 81

training guidelines, 165

training programs

advanced whole-body programs, 200

designing, 183-184

variables, 184

intensity, 185-187

periodization, 193-194

phases, 195-197

program cycles, 194-195

progression, 193-194

recovery, 191-192

sequence, 192-193

volume, 187-191

triple jumps, 176

trunk exercises

cable trunk rotation with press, 97

cable trunk rotation with pull, 96

flat bench, trunk flexion, 89

incline bench, trunk flexion, 87

seated trunk exercises, 94

supine trunk rotation, 95

Swiss ball, trunk flexion, 88

Swiss ball, trunk lateral flexion, 93

upper body exercises

barbell and bench, chest press, 132

barbell and bench, triceps press, 159

barbell lat row, 139

barbell scapular elevation, 149

cable, one-arm bicep flexion, 163

cable, one-arm decline press (lunge position), 134

cable, one-arm low lat row, 143

cable, one-arm low rear delt row, 148

cable, one-arm triceps extension, 158

cable, overhead bicep flexion, 162

cable, overhead lat row, 142

cable, overhead rear delt row, 147

cable, overhead triceps extension, 157

cable, seated lat pulldown, 144

cable, seated lat row, 141

cable, shoulder horizontal external rotation, 152

cable, shoulder horizontal internal rotation, 153

cable, shoulder integrated external rotation, 154

cable, shoulder integrated internal rotation, 155

dumbbell and bench, chest press, 130

dumbbell and bench, incline press, 135

dumbbell and Swiss ball, one-arm chest press, 131-132

dumbbell and Swiss ball, one-arm incline press, 136

dumbbell and Swiss ball, triceps extension, 156

dumbbell bicep flexion, 161

dumbbell one-arm lat row, 140

dumbbell rear delt row, 146

dumbbell, delt press (lunge position), 137

dumbbell, one-arm and -leg, delt press, 138
dumbbell, shoulder external rotation, 150
dumbbell, shoulder internal rotation, 151
machine, lat pull-up, 145
squat rack, pushup, 133
squat rack, triceps pushup, 160
X pattern, 171
exhaustion, 191
explosive-strength, 36
extensibility, joints, 40

F

fasciculi, 7
fast-twitch fibers, muscles, 46
fiber recruitment, strength, 34
fibers, muscles, 7, 34, 46
fibrocartilage, 6
fibrous joints, 3
figure eight pattern exercise, 172
flat bench exercises
    bent-leg hip flexion, 98
    trunk flexion, 89
flexibility, 40
forward overhand throw (med ball) exercise, 179
forward pass (med ball) exercise, 178
forward pullover throw (med ball) exercise, 179
forward underhand throw (med ball) exercise, 178
four-point core activation, resistance training, 80
frequency, training programs, 190
frontal plane (movement), 10
fusiform muscle-tendon unit, 7

G–H

Gambetta, Vern, 65
gamma motor neurons, spinal cord, 25-26
general coordination, 51
general motor pattern compatibility, 65
general plain motion, resistance training, 61

general training goals, resistance training, 58
glenoid fossa (shoulder socket), 62
glute kickers exercise, 166
Golgi tendon organs, 26

hang clean exercise, 181
hexagon jump pattern exercise, 177
high knees exercise, 166
horizontal plane (movement), 10
human movement systems, 2
    active (muscular) system, 6-10, 17-24
    control (sensorimotor) system, 24-30
    passive (skeleton) system, 3-6
hyaline cartilage, 6
hypertrophy phase (training programs), 196

I–J

impact stability demand, 38
incline bench exercises
    incline bench, trunk extension, 91
    straight-leg hip flexion, 99
    Swiss ball, trunk extension, 92
    Swiss ball, trunk lateral flexion, 93
    trunk flexion, 87
inclined bench exercises, double-leg hip extension, 101
initial volume (exercising), 187
inner unit (core), muscles, 19-21
intensity, training programs, 185-187
intermuscular coordination, 34
intramuscular coordination, 34
iso-kinetic exercises, tib flexion, 129
isolated joint kinematics, 9-10
isolated uniplanular joint muscles, 1
isometric contraction (muscles), 9

joint capsules, 6
joints, 3, 5
    biaxial joints, 5
    cartilaginous joints, 5

connective tissue, 5-6
extensibility, 40
fibrous joints, 3
isolated joint kinematics, 9-10
isolated uniplanular joint muscles, 1
stiffness, components, 40
synovial joints, 5
unilaxial joints, 5
Jones, Arthur, 73
jump and reach exercise, 173
jump and tuck exercise, 173
jump training, 54
jump with glute kick exercise, 174

K–L

kinematics (muscle), 1
kinesthesia, 72

lateral crossover run, 169
lateral jumps exercise, 176
lateral shuffle exercise, 168
lateral subsystem (LS), muscles, 23-24
lateral throw (med ball) exercise, 180
ligaments, 5, 63
linear motion, resistance training, 60
local muscular endurance, 36
long jumps (hops) exercise, 175
lower body exercises
    45-degree hip extension, 102
    balance squats, 108
    barbell dead lift, 112
    barbell hip extension, 103
    barbell squats, 111
    body weight squats, 107
    body weight, reverse lunge, 116
    body weight, stationary lunge, 114
    cable hip abduction, 105
    cable hip adduction, 106
    cable, ham flexion, 123
    cable, quad extension, 121
    dumbbell, narrow squats, 110
    dumbbell, one-leg calf extension, 125
    dumbbell, one-leg hip extension, 104

dumbbell, reverse lunge, 117
dumbbell, stationary lunge, 115
dumbbell, traveling lunge, 119
dumbbell, wide squats, 109
flat bench, bent-leg hip flexion, 98
incline bench, straight-leg hip flexion, 99
inclined bench, double-leg hip extension, 101
iso-kinetic tib flexion, 129
machine, bent-leg calf extension, 127
machine, calf extension, 126
machine, ham flexion, 124
machine, quad extension, 122
machine, seated leg press, 113
machine, tib flexion, 128
med ball, traveling lunge (side load), 120
Swiss ball, double-leg hip flexion, 100
traveling lunge, 118
lower body power exercises
hexagon jump pattern, 177
jump and reach, 173
jump and tuck, 173
jump with glute kick, 174
lateral jumps, 176
long jumps (hops), 175
lunge jump, 175
single-leg lateral jumps, 177
triple jumps, 176
lower brain, 26-27
LS (lateral subsystem), muscles, 23-24
lunge jump exercise, 175

M

machine exercises
bent-leg calf extension, 127
calf extension, 126
ham flexion, 124
lat pull-up, 145
quad extensions, 122
seated leg press, 113
tib flexion, 128

macrocycles, 194
maximal oxygen consumption (VO2 max), 36
maximal-strength, 35
maximal-strength phase (training programs), 196
mechanoreceptors, 26
median plane (movement), 10
medicine ball exercises
backward underhand throw, 180
forward overhand throw, 179
forward pass, 178
forward pullover throw, 179
forward underhand throw, 178
lateral throw, 180
traveling lunge (side load), 120
mobility
flexibility, 40
improving, 39-41
active stretching, 42
passive stretching, 41
passive-active stretching, 43
ROM (range of motion), 39-40
motor cortex, 28
motor learning, 28-30
motor programs, 72
motor responses, levels, 25-28
motor units, 25, 34
movement systems, 2
active (muscular) system, 6-10, 17-24
control (sensorimotor) system, 24-30
passive (skeleton) system, 3-6
muscle kinematics, 1
muscle spindles, 26
muscles
actions, 17-18
active insufficiency, 9
agonists, 17
antagonists, 17
fibers, types of, 46
fusiform muscle-tendon unit, 7
inner unit (core), 19-21
intermuscular coordination, 34
intramuscular coordination, 34
isolated uniplanular joint muscles, 1
local muscular endurance, 36
muscle fibers, 7
muscle kinematics, 1
neutralizers, 17

reciprocal inhibition, 17
roles, 17-18
skeletal muscles, 18
stabilizers, 17
synergists, 17
tendons, 7-8
muscular system (movement), 1, 6-10, 17-24
musculoskeletal system, 7
neuromuscular system, 7
subsystems, 19
anterior oblique subsystem (AOS), 23
deep longitudinal subsystem (DLS), 21-22
lateral subsystem (LS), 23-24
posterior oblique subsystem (POS), 22-23
musculoskeletal system, 7
resistance training, 59-60
myofibrils (muscle fiber), 7
myosin, 7
myotatic stretch reflexes, 54-55

N–O

narrow squats (dumbbell), 110
neural-metabolic continuum, adaptation to time under tension, 188
neurological considerations, resistance training, 59-60
neuromuscular coordination, agility, 51
neuromuscular efficiency, 28-30, 51, 72
neuromuscular system, 7
neurons
gamma motor neurons, 26
motor units, 25
neutralizers (muscles), 17
number encoding, intramuscular coordination, 34

OBLA (onset of blood lactate accumulation), 37
one-point core activation, resistance training, 84
onset of blood lactate accumulation (OBLA), 37
optimal posture, positioning, resistance training, 68-69
overtraining, 191

P

passive-flexibility, 40
passive stretching, 41
passive system (movement), 1-6
passive-active stretching, 43
path of motion, resistance training, 60-61
pattern encoding, intramuscular coordination, 34
pattern overloads, 191
perimysium, 7
periodization
    recommendations, 211-212
    training programs, 193-194
perpendicular planes (movement), 10
phases, training programs, 195-197
plain motion, resistance training, 61
planes (movement), 10
plyometrics, 54-55
PNF (Proprioceptive Neuromuscular Facilitation) stretching, 43
POS (posterior oblique subsystem), muscles, 22-23
positioning, resistance training, 67-70
    goals, 70
    optimal posture, 68-69
    spine, 67-68
posterior oblique subsystem (POS), muscles, 22-23, 143
posterior somatic sensory cortex, 28
posture, resistance training, 68-69
power
    deficit of, 54
    improving, 52-55
    myotatic stretch reflexes, 54-55
    plyometrics, 54-55
    prerequisites, 53-54
    training, 53, 55
power clean exercise, 181
power exercises
    lower body
        hexagon jump pattern, 177
        jump and reach, 173
        jump and tuck, 173

jump with glute kick, 174
lateral jumps, 176
long jumps (hops), 175
lunge jump, 175
single-leg lateral jumps, 177
triple jumps, 176
    upper body
        hang clean, 181
        med ball, backward underhand throw, 180
        med ball, forward overhand throw, 179
        med ball, forward pass, 178
        med ball, forward pullover throw, 179
        med ball, forward underhand throw, 178
        med ball, lateral throw, 180
        power clean, 181
        power pushups, 182
        push-press (jerk), 182
power phase (training programs), 197
power pushups, 182
power skipping exercise, 168
programs (training)
    advanced split programs, 202-210
    advanced whole-body programs, 199-200
    base programs, 197-198
    cycles, 194-195
    progression, 193-194
    recovery, 191-192
progression, training programs, 193-194
progressive dynamic stretching, 42
pronation, 10
Proprioceptive Neuromuscular Facilitation (PNF) stretching, 43
push-press (jerk) exercise, 182

Q–R

quadraplex, resistance training, 82
quickness, 47

range of motion (ROM), 39-40, 61
    resistance training, 61-65

rate encoding, intramuscular coordination, 34
reciprocal inhibition (muscles), 17
recovery, training programs, 191-192
recovery adjustments, intensity, 186
reflexes
    balance, 39
    body-righting, 71
    myotatic stretch, 54-55
    tilting-response, 71
relative-strength, 35
resistance training, 57-58
    alignment, 66-67
    breathing, 74-76
    exercise motion, 60-66
        path of motion, 60-61
        range of motion, 61-65
        type of motion, 60-61
    general training goals, 58
    musculoskeletal considerations, 59-60
    neurological considerations, 59-60
    overall goals, 58
    positioning, 67-70
        goals, 70
        optimal posture, 68-69
        spine, 67-68
    specific training goals, 58-59
    stabilization, 70-72
        balance, 71
        core function, 72
    stabilization exercises, 79
        four-point core activation, 80
        one-point core activation, 84
        quadraplex, 82
        standing core activation, 83
        supine core activation, 85-86
        two-point core activation, 81
    strength exercises, 79
        four-point core activation, 80
        one-point core activation, 84
        quadraplex, 82
        standing core activation, 83

supine core activation, 85-86
two-point core activation, 81
suggestions, 79
tempo, 72-74
assignments, 73-74
science of, 73
ROM (range of motion), 39-40
rotatory motion, resistance training, 60
running mechanics, 49-50

S

SAID (Specific Adaptations to the Imposed Demands) Principle, 53-54, 65
sarcomere (muscle fiber), 9
sensorimotor system (movement), 1, 24-30
motor responses, levels, 25-28
sequence, training programs, 192-193
shuttle run patterns exercise, 172
single-leg lateral jumps exercise, 177
skeletal muscles, 18
skeleton, 3-6
bone groups, 3-4
composition, 3-4
functions, 3
joints, 3-6
musculoskeletal system, 7
neuromuscular system, 7
slow-twitch fibers, muscles, 46
special coordination, 51
Specific Adaptations to the Imposed Demands (SAID) Principle. *See* SAID (Specific Adaptations to the Imposed Demands) Principle
specific coordination, 51
specific training goals, resistance training, 58-59
speed
agility, speed training, 52
exercises
backpedal plants with sprint, 170
backpedaling, 170

bounding, 167
carioca, 169
drum majors, 167
figure eight pattern, 172
glute kickers, 166
high knees, 166
lateral crossover run, 169
lateral shuffle, 168
power skipping, 168
shuttle run patterns, 172
square pattern, 171
X pattern, 171
improving, 46-50
quickness, 47
running mechanics, 49-50
strength, relationship, 47-48
speed-strength, 35
spinal cord, 25
positioning, resistance training, 67-68
split programs, 202-210
square pattern exercise, 171
squat exercises
balance squats, 108
barbell squats, 111
body weight squats, 107
dumbbell narrow squats, 110
dumbbell wide squats, 109
pushups, 133
triceps pushup, 160
stability
balance, 39
breathing, relationships, 76
dynamic stability, 70
dynamic stability demand, 38
improving, 38-39
static stability, 38, 70
stabilization exercises, 79
45-degree hip extension, 102
balance squats, 108
barbell and bench, chest press, 132
barbell hip extension, 103
barbell lat roll, 139
barbell lift, 112
barbell scapular elevation, 149
barbell squats, 111
body weight squats, 107
body weight, reverse lunge, 116
body weight, stationary lunge, 114
cable hip abduction, 105

cable hip adduction, 106
cable one-arm decline press (lunge position), 134
cable trunk rotation with press, 97
cable trunk rotation with pull, 96
cable, ham flexion, 123
cable, one-arm low lat row, 143
cable, one-arm low rear delt row, 148
cable one-arm bicep flexion, 163
cable one-arm triceps extension, 158
cable overhead bicep flexion, 162
cable, overhead lat row, 142
cable, overhead rear delt row, 147
cable overhead triceps extension, 157
cable, quad extension, 121
cable, seated lat pulldown, 144
cable, seated lat row, 141
cable, shoulder horizontal external rotation, 152
cable, shoulder horizontal internal rotation, 153
cable, shoulder integrated external rotation, 154
cable, shoulder integrated internal rotation, 155
core function, 72
dumbbell and bench, chest press, 130
dumbbell and bench, incline press, 135
dumbbell and Swiss ball, triceps extension, 156
dumbbell and Swiss ball, one-arm chest press, 131-132
dumbbell and Swiss ball, one-arm incline press, 136
dumbbell bicep flexion, 161
dumbbell, delt press (lunge position), 137
dumbbell one-arm lat row, 140
dumbbell rear delt row, 146
dumbbell, narrow squats, 110
dumbbell, one-arm and -leg delt press, 138

dumbbell, one-leg calf extension, 125

dumbbell, one-leg hip extension, 104

dumbbell, reverse lunge, 117

dumbbell, shoulder external rotation, 150

dumbbell, shoulder internal rotation, 151

dumbbell, stationary lunge, 115

dumbbell, traveling lunge, 119

dumbbell, wide squats, 109

flat bench, bent-leg hip flexion, 98

flat bench, trunk flexion, 89

four-point core activation, 80

incline bench, straight-leg hip flexion, 99

incline bench, trunk extension, 91

incline bench, trunk flexion, 87

inclined bench, double-leg hip extension, 101

iso-kinetic tib flexion, 129

machine, bent-leg calf extension, 127

machine, calf extension, 126

machine, ham flexion, 124

machine, lat pull-up, 145

machine, quad extension, 122

machine, seated leg press, 113

machine, tib flexion, 128

med ball, traveling lunge (side load), 120

one-point core activation, 84

quadraplex, 82

seated trunk exercises, 94

squat rack, pushup, 133

standing core activation, 83

supine core activation, 85-86

supine trunk rotation, 95

Swiss ball, double-leg hip flexion, 100

Swiss ball, reverse trunk flexion, 90

Swiss ball, trunk extension, 92

Swiss ball, trunk flexion, 88

Swiss ball, trunk lateral flexion, 93

traveling lunge, 118

two-point core activation, 81

kinesthesia, 72

motor programs, 72

resistance training, 70-72

squat rack, triceps pushup, 160

stabilizers (muscles), 17

standing core activation, resistance training, 83

starting-strength, 35

static stability, 38, 70

static-strength, 35

stiffness, joints, components, 40

strength

absolute, 35

acceleration, 35

core control, 53

endurance, 35, 53

exercises, 79

45-degree hip extension, 102

balance squats, 108

barbell and bench, chest press, 132

barbell and bench, triceps press, 159

barbell dead-lift, 112

barbell hip extension, 103

barbell lat roll, 139

barbell scapular elevation, 149

barbell squats, 111

body weight squats, 107

body weight, reverse lunge, 116

body weight, stationary lunge, 114

cable hip abduction, 105

cable hip adduction, 106

cable one-arm decline press (lunge position), 134

cable trunk rotation with press, 97

cable trunk rotation with pull, 96

cable, ham flexion, 123

cable, one-arm bicep flexion, 163

cable, one-arm low lat row, 143

cable, one-arm low rear delt row, 148

cable, one-arm triceps extension, 158

cable, overhead bicep flexion, 162

cable, overhead lat row, 142

cable, overhead rear delt row, 147

cable, overhead triceps extension, 157

cable, quad extension, 121

cable, seated lat pulldown, 144

cable, seated lat row, 141

cable, shoulder horizontal external rotation, 152

cable, shoulder horizontal internal rotation, 153

cable, shoulder integrated external rotation, 154

cable, shoulder integrated internal rotation, 155

dumbbell and bench, chest press, 130

dumbbell and bench, incline press, 135

dumbbell and Swiss ball, one-arm chest press, 131-132

dumbbell and Swiss ball, one-arm incline press, 136

dumbbell and Swiss ball, triceps extension, 156

dumbbell bicep flexion, 161

dumbbell one-arm lat row, 140

dumbbell rear delt row, 146

dumbbell, delt press (lunge position), 137

dumbbell, narrow squats, 110

dumbbell, one-arm and -leg, delt press, 138

dumbbell, one-leg calf extension, 125

dumbbell, one-leg hip extension, 104

dumbbell, reverse lunge, 117

dumbbell, shoulder external rotation, 150
dumbbell, shoulder internal rotation, 151
dumbbell, stationary lunge, 115
dumbbell, traveling lunge, 119
dumbbell, wide squats, 109
flat bench, bent-leg hip flexion, 98
flat bench, trunk flexion, 89
four-point core activation, 80
incline bench, straight-leg hip flexion, 99
incline bench, trunk extension, 91
incline bench, trunk flexion, 87
inclined bench, double-leg hip extension, 101
iso-kinetic tib flexion, 129
machine, bent-leg calf extension, 127
machine, calf extension, 126
machine, ham flexion, 124
machine, lat pull-up, 145
machine, quad extension, 122
machine, seated leg press, 113
machine, tib flexion, 128
med ball, traveling lunge (side load), 120
one-point core activation, 84
quadraplex, 82
seated trunk rotation, 94
squat rack, pushup, 133
squat rack, triceps pushup, 160
standing core activation, 83
supine core activation, 85-86
supine trunk rotation, 95
Swiss ball, double-leg hip flexion, 100

Swiss ball, reverse trunk flexion, 90
Swiss ball, trunk extension, 92
Swiss ball, trunk flexion, 88
Swiss ball, trunk lateral flexion, 93
traveling lunge, 118
two-point core activation, 81
explosive strength, 36
fiber recruitment, 34
improving, 33-36
intermuscular coordination, 34
intramuscular coordination, 34
maximal, 35
misconceptions, 34
motor units, 34
relative, 35
speed, 53
relationship, 47-48
speed, 35
starting, 35
static, 35
trunk, 53
stretching, 41-43
subsystems, muscles, 19
anterior oblique subsystem (AOS), 23
deep longitudinal subsystem (DLS), 21-22
lateral subsystem (LS), 23-24
posterior oblique subsystem (POS), 22-23
summation phases (power), 54
supercompensation, 191
supersetting, 192
supination, 10
supine core activation, resistance training, 85-86
Swiss ball exercises
double-leg hip flexion, 100
one-arm chest press, 131-132
one-arm incline press, 136
reverse trunk flexion, 90
triceps extension, 156
trunk flexion, 88
synergistic dominance (muscles), 17
synergists (muscles), 17
synovial joints, 5

T
tempo, resistance training, 72-74
tendons, 7-8
aponeurosis tendons, 20
Golgi tendon organs, 26
thoracolumbar fascia, 20
thoracolumbar fascia, tendons, 20
tilting-response reflexes, 39, 71
total volume (exercising), 187
training programs
advanced split programs, 202-210
advanced whole-body programs, 199-200
base program, 197-198
designing, 183-184
advanced whole-body programs, 200
intensity, 185-187
periodization, 193-194
phases, 195-197
program cycles, 194-195
progression, 193-194
recovery, 191-192
sequence, 192-193
variables, 184
volume, 187-191
periodization, recommendations, 211-212
transitional phase (training programs), 195
translatory motion, resistance training, 60
traveling lunge, 118
triple jumps exercise, 176
trunk exercises
cable trunk rotation with press, 97
cable trunk rotation with pull, 96
flat bench, trunk flexion, 89
incline bench, trunk extension, 91
incline bench, trunk flexion, 87
seated trunk exercises, 94
supine trunk rotation, 95
Swiss ball, reverse trunk flexion, 90
Swiss ball, trunk extension, 92
Swiss ball, trunk flexion, 88
Swiss ball, trunk lateral flexion, 93

trunk strength, 53

two-point core activation, resistance training, 81

type of motion, resistance training, 60-61

U

uniaxial joints, 5

uniplanular joint muscles, 1

upper body exercises

    barbell and bench, chest press, 132

    barbell and bench, triceps press, 159

    barbell lat roll, 139

    barbell scapular elevation, 149

    cable one-arm decline press (lunge position), 134

    cable, one-arm bicep flexion, 163

    cable, one-arm lat row, 143

    cable, one-arm low rear delt row, 148

    cable, one-arm triceps extension, 158

    cable, overhead bicep flexion, 162

    cable, overhead lat row, 142

    cable, overhead rear delt row, 147

    cable, overhead triceps extension, 157

    cable, seated lat pulldown, 144

    cable, seated lat row, 141

    cable, shoulder horizontal external rotation, 152

    cable, shoulder horizontal internal rotation, 153

    cable, shoulder integrated external rotation, 154

    cable, shoulder integrated internal rotation, 155

    dumbbell and bench, chest press, 130

    dumbbell and bench, incline press, 135

    dumbbell and Swiss ball, one-arm chest press, 131-132

    dumbbell and Swiss ball, one-arm incline press, 136

    dumbbell and Swiss ball, triceps extension, 156

    dumbbell bicep flexion, 161

    dumbbell one-arm lat row, 140

    dumbbell rear delt row, 146

    dumbbell, delt press (lunge press), 137

    dumbbell, one-arm and -leg, delt press, 138

    dumbbell, shoulder external rotation, 150

    dumbbell, shoulder internal rotation, 151

    machine, lat pull-up, 145

    squat rack, pushup, 133

    squat rack, triceps pushup, 160

upper body power exercises

    hang clean, 181

    med ball, backward underhand throw, 180

    med ball, forward overhand throw, 179

    med ball, forward pass, 178

    med ball, forward pullover throw, 179

    med ball, forward underhand throw, 178

    med ball, lateral throw, 180

    power clean, 181

    power pushups, 182

    push-press (jerk), 182

V–W–X–Y–Z

Valsalva Maneuver, exercise breathing, 75

Verkhoshansky, Yuri, 54

VO2 max (maximal oxygen consumption), 36

volume, training programs, 186-191

whole-body programs, 199-200

wide squats (dumbbell), 109

X pattern exercise, 171